INDOOR POLLUTION

INDOOR POLLUTION

Steve Coffel and Karyn Feiden

FAWCETT COLUMBINE • NEW YORK

A Fawcett Columbine Book
Published by Ballantine Books
Copyright © 1990 by Steve Coffel and Karyn Feiden
Illustrations copyright © by Random House, Inc.

Library of Congress Catalog Card Number: 90-82343

ISBN: 0-449-90476-8

Cover design by Dale Fiorillo
Manufactured in the United States of America
First Edition: January 1991
10 9 8 7 6 5 4 3 2 1

CONTENTS

ACKNOWLEDGMENTS

Special thanks to our editor, Lynn Rosen, for her care and interest in this project, and to our agent and favorite deal-maker, Barbara Lowenstein of Lowenstein Associates. Our gratitude also goes to the New York Committee on Occupational Safety and Health (NYCOSH) for the generosity with which they opened their files to us in the course of our research—as well as for their longstanding commitment to worker health and safety.

INDOOR POLLUTION

1
AN OVERVIEW

Notions about the sanctity of home run deep in literature, religion, and philosophy. "What is more agreeable than one's home?" asked the Roman orator Cicero, a sentiment seconded in Sir Edward Coke's oft-quoted statement: "A man's house is his castle." Much more recently, Dorothy was sent spinning back to Kansas from the Land of Oz by chanting: "There's no place like home, there's no place like home, there's no place like home."

But scientists are discovering that our homes may not actually be the safe and secure places we have long assumed. In fact, some alarming research suggests that the air inside American houses and apartments is dangerously polluted by a toxic mix of chemicals, airborne fibers, and biological invaders.

Sound bad? There is no running to the workplace to escape. Windows that won't open, malfunctioning exhaust and ventilation systems, and the absence of circulating outdoor air allow contaminants from office equipment, building materials, furnishings, and cigarettes to build to unsafe levels. What office workers describe as "the bug that's going around" may actually be the effects of these accumulated toxic substances.

The severity of indoor pollution comes into even sharper focus when concern about drinking water is considered. Thousands of substances used in industrial and agricultural processes, including gasoline, radioactive materials, chemicals, pesticides, heavy metals, and biological agents, can contaminate the lakes, rivers, streams, and aquifers that supply

3

household water. Despite elaborate treatment and process-ing—and sometimes because of them—the safeguards in place in most communities are simply insufficient to guarantee pure drinking water.

Because indoor pollution is generally invisible to the eye and its effects on human health may not be apparent for many years, it is hard to assess the true hazards of contami-nation. But disquieting irritations, rashes, congestion, fa-tigue, some childhood respiratory diseases, and cancer have all been associated with toxic substances in our homes and workplaces. The Consumer Federation of America, a con-sumer protection group headquartered in Washington, D.C., calls indoor air pollution the nation's number one hidden health threat.

Unfortunately, a sense of urgency has yet to surround the problem. In the 1970s, public and legislative attention began to be focused on the *outdoor* environment. But effective pub-lic policies to improve the *indoor* environment remain in their infancy. Heightening public awareness about indoor pollu-tion and making the legislative and policy changes that will assure safe and decent housing and a workplace free of con-tamination have become imperative.

There are still no uniform standards to define safe con-centration levels of specific contaminants in the home. No single federal agency has been charged with overseeing all of the government's indoor air and water quality activities. And the public and private resources allocated to research and public education in the field have been clearly inadequate.

In the workplace, the standards set by the Occupational Safety and Health Administration (OSHA) and other federal regulatory agencies are generally targeted at industrial plants, where chemicals are often used at very high concentrations. Although worker protection in such environments may be inadequate, at least some safeguards for limiting toxic expo-sure do exist. By contrast, exposure to the hazards of office buildings—from photocopiers and office supplies to newly in-

stalled carpeting and excess moisture—is virtually unregu-
lated.

Solutions to the problems of indoor pollution do exist.
Along with an in-depth look at the hazards of contaminated
air and water, this book offers concrete, practical, and af-
fordable ways of dealing with them. Making wise decisions
when buying household furnishings or cleaning products, undertaking building renovations cautiously, installing simple
pollution control devices, and keeping relative humidity levels low are just a few modest steps that have an enormous
impact on human health and comfort.

Indoor Pollution also explores the political arena, arguing
that homeowners and apartment dwellers, legislators and
public policymakers, employees and employers, product
manufacturers and commercial building operators all have
roles to play in creating a healthy environment for living and
working. A sample letter you can write to a legislator is included in the Appendix to aid you in taking an active role in
combating the problems of indoor pollution.

WHAT CAUSES INDOOR POLLUTION?

The problems of indoor pollution are not new. In fact, the
first known incident dates back to the days when human beings were still living in caves. Once these early people discovered the warmth of fire, soot became encrusted on the
roof of primitive shelters—an indication that inadequate ventilation had allowed carbon monoxide and other gases to accumulate.

Some more recent examples:

- A group of Oregon homemakers between the ages of
  sixteen and sixty-four were studied for fifteen years and
  found to be twice as likely to die of cancer as working women. The blame is being placed on chronic ex-

posure to the carcinogens contained in many cleaning
materials.

- Dozens of children living on an Indian reservation along
  Maine's majestic coastline are suffering from respiratory illnesses. The tightly sealed, energy-efficient
  homes built for their families by the federal government in the early 1970s are the likely source of the
  problem.

- Carbon monoxide levels in the kitchens of some well-
  insulated homes are three times greater than the concentration in the car-crazy metropolis of Los Angeles.

- Chemical sensitivities have forced a Harvard Law
  School student into a tent to avoid indoor pesticide poisoning, confined a Philadelphia woman to one room in
  her house, and incapacitated a Michigan man after he
  was exposed to vapors emitting from a waterproofing
  compound, according to anecdotes documented by the
  National Center for Environmental Health Strategies.

- Ironically, serious workplace problems surfaced inside
  the central headquarters of the Environmental Protection Agency (EPA) in Washington, D.C., where contamination made more than 100 people ill. Several EPA
  employees who were able to tolerate visits to outdoor
  hazardous waste sites felt sick after only fifteen minutes in the office.

Two recent developments explain most indoor pollution
problems: the growing use of chemicals and synthetic materials and the push toward more tightly sealed homes and office buildings.

The Sources of Pollution

Ordinary living is a dirty business, at least as far as air
quality is concerned. An average family of four vaporizes 4
to 10 gallons of water a day in the process of cooking, breathing, and sweating. In tightly insulated homes without adequate ventilation, humidity levels are sent soaring,

encouraging the growth of molds and fungi and damaging a home's windowsills, furnishings, and wooden structural elements. Human beings also exhale carbon dioxide, ammonia, acetone, ketone, hydrogen chloride, nitrogen dioxide, methane, and a host of other potentially toxic substances, as well as a variety of virulent microorganisms.

The problems created when this biologically derived air becomes trapped are intensified by the growing use of synthetics and chemicals in construction materials, home furnishings, plastics, cleaning products, aerosol sprays, and scores of other common household products. Particleboard cabinetry and some fabrics* emit formaldehyde, while volatile organic chemicals evaporate from common cleaning and personal care products, as well as from drinking and bathing water. At the same time, asbestos fibers hover unseen in the air. Even seemingly innocuous house dust can be unwholesome, since it contains dry flakes from skin and hair, mites, and the many hazardous substances found in cigarette smoke.

Nor do the problems end there. Conventional heating and cooking sources spew out poisonous gas, and a lengthy list of contaminants can seep in from outside. Radon is the best-known of these, but emissions from an upwind industrial plant or the neighbor's wood stove, automobile exhaust from an attached garage, pesticides, biological agents, and dust particles laden with heavy metals from nearby roadways can also create health hazards. If you are unlucky enough to live near toxic wastes or the site of a chemical spill, poisonous vapors may add to this lethal brew.

Many everyday household products contribute more than one toxic substance to the air. Synthetic wall-to-wall carpeting is a good example. When first installed, it emits formaldehyde fumes and numerous other toxic chemicals, including ethyl benzene, toluene, xylene, and styrene. The glues used

---

*Fabrics used in drapery, upholstery, and carpeting can contain urea-formaldehyde resins. Permanent-press cloth used for clothing also emits formaldehyde.

to secure the carpeting also emit toxics as they cure. Within a month or so, most of the offending chemicals have been released, but aging then introduces its own hazards. Carpet fibers become brittle as they weather, adding to airborne dust. And the difficulties of thoroughly cleaning wall-to-wall carpeting means that it can harbor nutrients and moisture that become home to literally millions of microorganisms.

Many of the same dangers exist in the workplace, where additional sources of toxics can be found, particularly faulty ventilation systems and common office equipment, including photocopiers. "We have come to realize that we find pollutants in every building; and that indoor air pollution varies considerably by season, by building age, by type of heating, by the appliances you find in a building, by ventilation, by the products in use, and by the personal habits of the occupants," EPA Deputy Administrator A. James Barnes told a congressional subcommittee investigating the health hazards of indoor pollution.

The Hazards of Tightly Sealed Buildings

If outdoor air circulated freely through our homes and offices, it could purge the air of many toxic synthetics and eliminate much of the indoor pollution problem. Years ago, this principle was widely recognized, and windows and doors were commonly left ajar to reduce the risks of tuberculosis and other contagious diseases. A belief in the healthy properties of fresh air, coupled with the drafty construction techniques and materials of the day, meant a veritable gale whistled through most homes. Cheap fuel oil, natural gas, and electricity made it possible for Americans to continue this tradition of abundant ventilation without giving the subject much thought.

Until the mid-1970s, that is. Suddenly, fossil fuel prices shot through the roof. Fears mounted that the United States would be held hostage by OPEC, the cartel of oil-producing nations. President Jimmy Carter declared that the nation was engaged in "the moral equivalent of war," and the race was on to reduce consumption of fossil fuels.

Because buildings consume one-third of the nation's energy resources, energy-saving techniques for heating and cooling homes were billed not only as money savers but as acts of patriotism. Weatherization—the process of curbing the flow of outdoor air through the house—came into vogue. Homeowners were encouraged to seal building cracks, install weather stripping around windows and doors, and add wall insulation. Innovative construction techniques in superinsulated buildings went even further—sometimes, heat loss dropped so low that body heat alone could supply as much as one-fourth of a home's total heating needs, even in a severe climate. At the same time, and for the same reasons, the trend toward constructing commercial office buildings without operable windows accelerated, and the rate at which fresh outdoor air was introduced through ventilation systems was slashed.

Weatherization has achieved its desired goal. In a typically leaky house, the air is likely to be completely replaced two or more times each hour by fresh outdoor air. By contrast, only 10 percent—sometimes considerably less—of the air in a very tightly sealed building is exchanged every hour. But in the race to insulate, traditional maxims about the benefits of fresh air have been largely forgotten. Today, we are discovering that the trend toward increasingly tight buildings has a dark side.

Without the benefits of dilution from the outside, hazardous by-products of ordinary household activities can quickly build to toxic levels. Consider the costly lesson conservationists learned in Mt. Airy, Maryland, where a brick home intended as a model of energy efficiency was constructed. Heavy insulation, plastic sheeting, magnetic weather stripping, and leakproof windows reduced heat loss so dramatically that builders boasted it could be heated with a hair dryer. But toasty warm though it was, the building could not be occupied. As the circulation of outdoor air plummeted, formaldehyde gas levels shot up, radioactivity soared to 100 times the outdoor measure, and a gray-green mold appeared inside the windows.

Tightening a home or office to conserve energy doesn't cause indoor pollution problems, of course. But it does trap contaminants that could otherwise escape through windows, doors, and cracks in the building envelope. Fortunately, there need not be a backlash against energy conservation or a re-

---

How Tightening Your House Reduces Air Exchange Rates

Energy conservation measures don't cause pollution problems, but they can exacerbate them by slashing the rate at which indoor air is exchanged for outdoor air. Here's how air exchange rates fall as you tighten up your home:

House-Tightening Measure	Air Exchange Rate Reduction
Using storm windows or weather-stripping windows	6 percent
Weather-stripping doors	1 percent
Caulking	3 percent
Adding blown-in wall insulation	10 percent
Sealing ducts	9 percent
Total Reduction	29 percent

SOURCE: Bonneville Power Administration, Residential Weatherization Program, October 1984.

turn to the days when the nation's precious natural resources were thoughtlessly squandered. With proper planning, the careful use of appropriate technology, and a concerted commitment of resources, it is possible instead to meet the twin goals of conservation and good indoor air.

WHAT ARE THE HEALTH EFFECTS?

Sometimes specific health effects, such as headaches, eye irritation, skin rashes, sore throat, or a chronic cough, can be traced easily to one or more indoor pollutants. For example, carbon monoxide from an automobile idling in an attached garage can translate directly into headaches and fatigue. An asthma attack may be provoked by pollen from mold growing inside an interior wall dampened by a leak. When the irritant is removed—or the susceptible individual leaves the affected indoor space—the symptoms quickly fade.

Tragically, the effects of many other toxic substances are unknown or not immediately apparent. Some 50,000 to 60,000 chemicals are in regular use in American industry, and most have never been tested for toxicity in human beings. Low-level, long-term exposure to certain chemicals (such as benzene), radioactive materials (such as radon's decay products), or minute particles (such as asbestos) is insidious, generally producing no symptoms for two or three decades and then manifesting as cancer.

Scientists are also taking a hard look at the differences between low-level, chronic exposure and acute, short-term exposure to common contaminants. Historically, researchers have studied the effects of acute exposure to a single pollutant. But few of us are likely to linger long enough in the direct path of smokestack emissions to breathe a toxic dose of sulfur dioxide. Unless you are a miner, you will not be exposed to radon at anywhere near the standard allowed by the U.S. Mines Safety and Health Administration, which is roughly four times the EPA's maximum recommended residential level.

Also of concern is the cumulative effect of prolonged contact with low levels of a mix of contaminants. "What we don't have is the understanding of how these mixtures combine in the body in terms of producing an overall health effect. Sometimes we believe they're additive; sometimes we believe they're synergistic—in other words, more than additive—and sometimes they're antagonistic," says Erich Bretthauer of the EPA. But the information we do have is already cause for alarm. For example, smokers face *fifty times* the average risk of contracting cancer due to inhaled asbestos, as well as greater risks from radon exposure. More research about the health consequences of multiple contaminant exposure is a clear priority.

The health effects of indoor air pollution on certain high-risk groups are also chilling. Experts at the National Center for Environmental Health Strategies say that some particularly sensitive individuals have had to make radical lifestyle changes to avoid incapacitating illness. At its worst, they say, "indoor pollutants have produced a population of environmental refugees, some living as though under house arrest, their homes stripped of many furnishings and consumer products; others living nomadic lifestyles, a few in specially built trailers but most in stripped-down mobile homes, in cars, in vans, tents, or sheds, isolated from interaction with society and unable to earn a living or obtain many of the basic necessities of life."

Typically, children and the elderly are exposed to higher-than-average levels of indoor toxins because they spend so much time at home, yet their resistance to pollutants is often weak. Children are more vulnerable because they weigh less and their bodies are still developing, while older people are often grappling with chronic diseases and the consequences of a less efficient immune system. Pregnant and breastfeeding women, chemically sensitive people, smokers, and heavy drinkers are also more prone to the effects of airborne toxics. Anyone with another illness or an allergy faces heightened risks, and an individual taking medication is more susceptible to dangerous chemical interactions.

It will most likely be years before we are sure how much exposure to which contaminants pose a clear problem. But one somber fact is irrefutable: Millions of Americans are un-

---

Is the Air in Your Home Contaminated?

Sometimes pollution makes the air inside your home smell stale or pungent, but more often there's no way to detect the presence of contaminants through the senses. If you suspect that residential pollution is causing health problems, keep a log of the symptoms exhibited by members of your household.

Chances are, you could be breathing contaminated air if the answer to one or more of these questions is yes:

- Does more than one person in the same household display similar symptoms of illness?
- Do the people who are most often at home exhibit the most severe symptoms?
- Do visitors complain of irritation or illness after they have been in your home?
- Do symptoms vanish when affected individuals are away from the indoor space?
- Do the symptoms wax and wane with the seasons?
- Are the symptoms more severe when the windows of your home are closed?
- Did the symptoms begin after you moved into a new home or remodeled an old one? After you purchased new furnishings or added new insulation?

knowingly living and working under a toxic cloud of stagnant, poisoned air that can make them ill. "We cannot defer decision making for fifty years until we have all the health data," observes Dr. James E. Woods, Jr., a professor of building construction at Virginia Polytechnic Institute. In a society whose cancer rates are among the highest in the world, we ignore the growing problem of indoor pollution at our peril.

CIGARETTE SMOKING AND INDOOR POLLUTION

No overview of indoor pollution is complete without a close scrutiny of the contamination created by cigarette smoke. Despite the well-known health consequences of smoking, more than 25 percent of the adult population in the United States continues to indulge in a habit that former Surgeon General C. Everett Koop calls as addictive as heroin. Smoking, the largest single preventable cause of premature death and disability in the United States, has been definitively linked to lung cancer, emphysema, bronchitis, and heart disease. More than a thousand people die every day from tobacco-related illnesses.

An understanding of the effects of passive smoking is much more recent. Both at home and in the workplace, we now know that nonsmokers who are forced to breathe air polluted by cigarettes—whether from smoldering cigarettes or a smoker's exhalations—also place their health in jeopardy. Contaminants from environmental tobacco smoke have been found on the walls, furniture, and other surfaces almost anywhere that people smoke, especially in tightly insulated buildings. And nicotine, carbon monoxide, formaldehyde, ammonia, hydrocyanic acid, and numerous other chemical poisons have all been isolated in the saliva, blood, and urine of nonsmokers.

The pathbreaking 1986 Surgeon General's report, "The Health Consequences of Involuntary Smoking," brought the issue of passive smoking to the foreground of public aware-ness. That report concluded:

- Involuntary smoking is a cause of disease, including lung cancer, in healthy nonsmokers.
- The children of parents who smoke have more respi-ratory infections and other symptoms of respiratory disease, as well as slightly smaller increases in lung function as the lung matures, than children of non-smoking parents.
- Separating smokers and nonsmokers within the same air space may reduce, but does not eliminate, the ex-posure of nonsmokers to environmental tobacco smoke.

By confirming the suspicion that cigarette smoke pollutes indoor air, the Surgeon General's report provides important ammunition in the struggle to establish the rights of non-smokers. Segregating smokers from nonsmokers in the work-place, requiring restaurants to set aside no-smoking sections, and banning cigarettes altogether from airport terminals, trains, retail stores, and medical waiting rooms may be the single most important step policymakers can take to elimi-nate indoor toxics.

USING THIS BOOK

Armed with the knowledge of indoor air and water qual-ity problems that is provided in this book and equipped with the tools to overcome them, consumers, homeowners, ten-ants, and workers can do much to create healthier indoor environments. Providing adequate ventilation at home and at work is one major step toward reducing the concentration of contaminants—good air circulation keeps indoor humidity levels low and helps to pull potentially toxic substances out of the building. Effective ventilation devices, including air-to-air heat exchangers, heat pump ventilators, and exhaust vents, are all described in detail here.

But ventilation can't remove all pollutants. Where feasible, *source control* is recommended as the best way to reduce toxic emissions. Homeowners can readily plan renovations or new construction with air and water quality in mind. Choosing an appropriate water filtration system, erecting barriers against radon, sealing or removing products that emit toxic chemicals or release asbestos fibers, fine-tuning the stove to reduce emissions of carbon monoxide and nitrogen dioxide, and using safe building materials are other relatively easy ways to reduce pollution in private houses.

Even if you don't own a house, there is plenty you can do about indoor residential pollution. Many of the solutions described here are within a renter's control. Once you understand how synthetic materials contaminate the air, you can purchase nontoxic carpeting, curtains, upholstery, and furniture. It is seldom difficult to eliminate the moisture that breeds biological contamination or to move containers of paint, shellac, pesticides, or fuel to a storage area separated from your living space. While mechanical ventilation problems usually can be solved only by a landlord or building manager, sometimes all that needs to be done to improve ventilation is to crack open a few windows. If the problem is more complex, organizing an effective tenant group may give you the clout to get the necessary maintenance or repair work done.

As a worker, you may have more command over your environment than you realize. While you may not have a say in running the building's ventilation system, purchasing furniture, or arranging office renovations, there is much that informed and organized employees can do. Bringing in plants, lobbying for smoke-free sections and professional asbestos removal, finding out whether adequate fresh air is being introduced into the ventilation system, and insisting that ventilation equipment be maintained properly are all concrete ways to safeguard your own health and that of your fellow workers.

Part I of this book, *At Home*, provides detailed information about the sources of indoor air and water pollution, the associated health hazards, how to test for contamination, and ways to reduce or eliminate it. Chapter 2 looks at the synthetic toxic substances created by our industrial society, concentrating especially on asbestos, formaldehyde, and volatile organic compounds. Chapter 3 examines pollutants that originate from natural sources, notably radon and biological agents, while Chapter 4 focuses on combustion by-products. In Chapter 5, the science of ventilation is described in clear terms, and Chapter 6 examines the poisoning of our drinking water and what can be done about it.

Part II, *At Work*, looks at the growing problems of sick office buildings, how they affect worker health, and ways to cure them. Chapter 7 details the sources of indoor pollution in the workplace, with a special look at the faulty ventilation systems that plague so many public buildings. Chapter 8 emphasizes solutions, beginning with the need to identify the nature and sources of employee discomfort and moving on to explain how chemical and biological contamination can be controlled.

Part III, *Public Policy*, makes concrete recommendations for getting federal, state, and local governments, as well as the private sector, involved in solving the problems of indoor pollution. Chapter 9 urges consumers to educate and organize themselves to become an effective voice for change.

Finally, a detailed Appendix describes relevant federal environmental legislation; lists public and private agencies involved with indoor pollution; provides sources for testing equipment, ventilation devices, safe building materials, non-polluting household products, and air and water purifiers. There is also an extensive bibliography, a glossary, and two indexes. The handy checklist on page 268 will help you locate specific information quickly.

PART I:
AT HOME

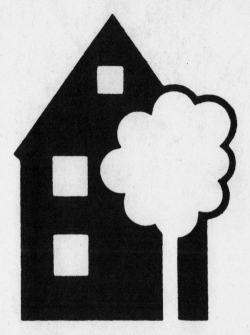

2
THE BY-PRODUCTS
OF AN INDUSTRIAL AGE
Asbestos, Formaldehyde, and
Volatile Organic Compounds

Many of the synthetic products in everyday use enhance the comfort and convenience of modern-day living. But the household products we take for granted—including appliances, furnishings, even cosmetics—often emit toxic substances or poisonous fibers into the air. Indeed, there are said to be more chemicals in the typical household today than in a well-equipped chemistry laboratory of a century ago. These chemicals can build to levels five to seventy times higher than outside the home, according to the Environmental Protection Agency, and extract punishing health and safety costs in the process.

As we begin our in-depth discussion of the hazards of specific contaminants, take heart. We also present practical solutions that will not unduly tax the budget or ingenuity of anyone who lives in a house or an apartment. Here's a closer look at asbestos, formaldehyde, and a range of gaseous contaminants known as volatile organic compounds, all of which originate from synthetic materials.

ASBESTOS

The word *asbestos* is derived from the Greek for "inextinguishable" and its use dates to ancient times. The Roman naturalist Pliny the Elder writes of shrouds woven from asbestos and wrapped around the bodies of nobility during cremation. Because it could not be consumed by fire, an asbestos lamp wick was often placed in temples consecrated to virgins, there to provide perpetual light. It is also said that flam-

21

boyant youths of olden days, perhaps eager to impress members of the opposite sex, sometimes covered themselves with asbestos cloth and walked through fire.

Since the dawn of the Industrial Revolution, the commercial value of asbestos has been widely recognized. Mined from the veins of metamorphic rock, the fibers are extraordinarily fine, strong, and flexible. A single pound of asbestos can yield six miles of silky fiber with a strength equivalent to certain kinds of steel and the ability to withstand temperatures approaching 400°C. The material is also waterproof, resistant to friction and corrosion, and sound absorbent.

In the course of the twentieth century, some 3,000 different products have been manufactured with the fibrous material. Around the world, asbestos use has jumped from 200,000 tons in 1920, to one million tons in 1950, to a staggering five million tons by the mid-1980s. Asbestos has been used to provide heat, acoustical insulation, and fireproofing, to strengthen building materials and make them more durable, to enhance the aesthetic value of a product, and even to make it easier to clean.

Asbestos insulation and fireproofing is most likely to be found in buildings constructed before the 1950s, especially in cold climates, where asbestos was wrapped around hot water pipes, steam pipes, furnaces, and boilers, and sprayed onto ceilings and walls as thermal and acoustic insulation or as a decorative finish. In one large Manhattan apartment building, a woman discovered asbestos when she was repainting the window trim in her four-year-old son's bedroom; she alerted her neighbors, who subsequently found asbestos chipping off the radiator and on pipes running through the closet. Most resilient floor tiles also contain asbestos, and the product is currently used in numerous household appliances, including refrigerators, dishwashers, ovens, and toasters.

Asbestos fibers can also be found

- In gypsum wallboard, textured paint, joint compound, and spackling compounds in homes built before the 1970s.

- In siding shingles and sheet flooring, especially in homes built during the 1950s. Asbestos is also found in floor tiles, a use that continues to this day.
- Sprayed onto walls and ceilings. Beginning in the 1930s, irregular surface areas were commonly sprayed with asbestos for decorative purposes or to provide acoustic insulation.
- Sprayed onto the steel supports of multistory buildings to protect them from warping as the result of fire, especially during the 1950s.
- Spun or woven into textiles, blankets, curtains, ropes, and lamp wicks and added to brake linings and automobile clutches, principally because of its value as fireproofing.

What Are the Health Hazards?

Despite the lengthy list of valuable uses, the miracle of the modern era has turned out to be a deadly hazard. An association between asbestos and disease was first observed in a French textile mill at the turn of the century; over the years, reports of lung disease among miners and other asbestos workers have mounted.

The dangers of asbestos have since been well established, and many building materials that contain the product were banned during the 1970s. Despite government restrictions aimed at barring the manufacture of all asbestos products by 1997, however, most of us are still surrounded by the product. It will be many decades before asbestos is eliminated altogether.

Fortunately, asbestos is dangerous only when the fibers are airborne. This happens as asbestos products age and become friable, or crumbly, or when they are disturbed, such as during renovation or demolition. Do-it-yourselfers who are unaware that a product in their home contains asbestos may accidentally dislodge the particles into the air in the process of cutting, scraping, or sanding a material. Hundreds of thousands of microscopic fibers can become suspended in each cubic foot of air inside any building with an asbestos problem.

Once asbestos fibers are inhaled, they can accumulate to toxic levels in the lungs. Known as silent killers because their devastating effects may not be evident until decades after exposure, asbestos fibers have been linked conclusively with asbestosis, a scarring of the lungs; mesothelioma, a rare cancer of the lining of the lung or abdomen; and uterine or gastrointestinal cancer.

Most asbestos-related diseases have been identified among individuals who work directly with the fibers, and it is clear that risk soars with frequency and intensity of exposure. The Occupational Safety and Health Administration (OSHA) limits workplace exposure to an average of no more than 0.2 fibers per cubic centimeter of air during an eight-hour period.

While no residential-level asbestos standards have been determined, experts agree that there is no safe threshold of asbestos exposure—in a worst-case scenario, even a single fiber lodged in just the wrong way has the potential to cause cancer. A few years ago, for example, a thirty-year-old man died of mesothelioma. Although he had never worked with asbestos, the man had grown up two blocks from the Brooklyn Navy Yard, where it was widely used in shipbuilding, and investigators concluded that fibers had become lodged in his lungs when he was a boy.

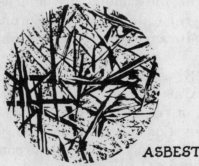

ASBESTOS FIBER

SOURCES OF ASBESTOS

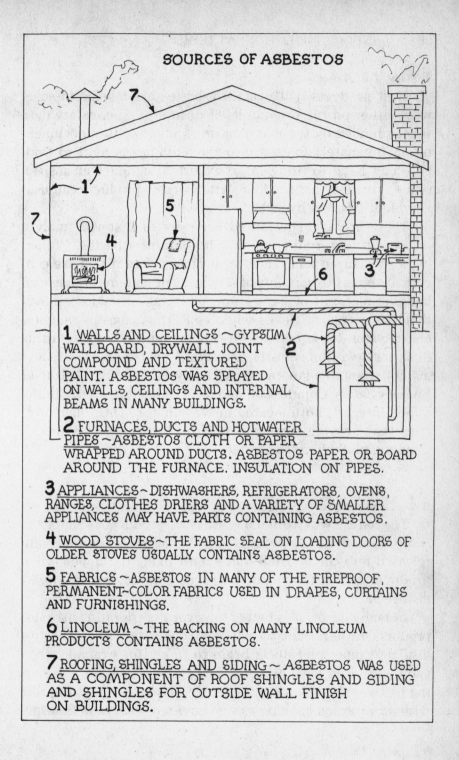

1 WALLS AND CEILINGS ~GYPSUM WALLBOARD, DRYWALL JOINT COMPOUND AND TEXTURED PAINT. ASBESTOS WAS SPRAYED ON WALLS, CEILINGS AND INTERNAL BEAMS IN MANY BUILDINGS.

2 FURNACES, DUCTS AND HOTWATER PIPES ~ASBESTOS CLOTH OR PAPER WRAPPED AROUND DUCTS. ASBESTOS PAPER OR BOARD AROUND THE FURNACE. INSULATION ON PIPES.

3 APPLIANCES ~ DISHWASHERS, REFRIGERATORS, OVENS, RANGES, CLOTHES DRIERS AND A VARIETY OF SMALLER APPLIANCES MAY HAVE PARTS CONTAINING ASBESTOS.

4 WOOD STOVES ~ THE FABRIC SEAL ON LOADING DOORS OF OLDER STOVES USUALLY CONTAINS ASBESTOS.

5 FABRICS ~ ASBESTOS IN MANY OF THE FIREPROOF, PERMANENT-COLOR FABRICS USED IN DRAPES, CURTAINS AND FURNISHINGS.

6 LINOLEUM ~ THE BACKING ON MANY LINOLEUM PRODUCTS CONTAINS ASBESTOS.

7 ROOFING, SHINGLES AND SIDING ~ ASBESTOS WAS USED AS A COMPONENT OF ROOF SHINGLES AND SIDING AND SHINGLES FOR OUTSIDE WALL FINISH ON BUILDINGS.

Testing for Asbestos

Most products that contain asbestos are labeled in some way, either on the product itself or in a product safety data sheet supplied by the manufacturer. Since written documentation for materials used in older buildings is hard to find, you may have to bring in an expert to conduct an inspection—a professional familiar with asbestos products can usually identify them by sight.

There are also specialized laboratories that will analyze material to determine whether it contains asbestos. Obtaining a specialized analysis is most appropriate if you are concerned about the contents of a significant amount of damaged building material or before you undertake a major renovation. Wear rubber gloves when collecting asbestos samples, and moisten loose chips with a plant mister before putting them inside a film canister or a tightly sealed plastic bag and mailing them to a laboratory for analysis. The U.S. Consumer Product Safety Commission and the Center for Science in the Public Interest, both located in Washington, D.C., have hotlines that provide further details on how to take a proper sampling and where to send it.

Asbestos Removal

The safest way to handle asbestos products is simply to leave them alone. Asbestos is only dangerous when fibers are released into the air, and that's most likely to happen when products are cut, drilled, scraped, sanded, or otherwise disturbed.

In many cases, it is better to cover deteriorating asbestos products rather than to attempt removal. When asbestos-insulated pipes and ducts begin to flake, for example, they can be covered with protective tape and sealed with a coating or two of latex paint. Similarly, damaged vinyl flooring with an asbestos backing can be covered with new flooring.

Wood, aluminum, or vinyl siding can be laid over asbestos siding, or spray paint can be used to seal in the asbestos fibers.

If you do have to remove asbestos products altogether, it is far safer to hire a contractor experienced with handling asbestos than to attempt the job yourself. Many states require accreditation of asbestos-removal specialists; a state or city environmental agency usually can provide lists of qualified contractors. Seek at least two estimates before agreeing to have asbestos removed and ask for a written quote, a list of the asbestos-containing materials to be removed, references, a work history, and a copy of an insurance certificate.

Whether you remove the asbestos yourself or hire a contractor to do the job, it is absolutely essential that appropriate precautions be taken, or you can worsen your problems rather than solve them. Here are some guidelines:

- Before beginning asbestos removal, the area should be isolated with a floor-to-ceiling plastic barrier secured with duct tape. A piece of plastic sheeting should be laid on the floor, and the entire space must be ventilated to the outside. Be particularly careful that asbestos-containing dust is not tracked into other parts of the house during the removal process.
- Anyone removing asbestos should wear an approved mask specifically designed for the purpose, a hat, and protective clothing that leaves no skin exposed to the air. Disposable rubbers, gloves, and coveralls are all available at local hardware stores. If possible, all clothing should be discarded once the job is completed. If you must wash material that has been exposed to asbestos dust, be sure to separate it from other laundry.
- To prevent fibers from becoming airborne, spray asbestos surfaces with a plant mister or a spray painter filled with water and adjusted to its finest setting until they are thoroughly damp, but not soaking wet. Adding one

teaspoon of low-sudsing dish or laundry detergent to a
quart of water increases penetration and reduces the
amount of water needed.

• Every effort should be made to remove asbestos materials without breaking them up any more than necessary. Asbestos-board panels, asbestos cloth and paper
are generally cut or broken into sections with metal
shears or heavy scissors. Rigid pipe wrap is usually cut
where the two halves have been taped together. Asbestos blown onto pipes, ceilings, and walls is usually
cut down to the surface on which it has been applied
and removed in sections. After the bulk of the material
has been removed, any residue is thoroughly scraped
and sponged off.

• Once asbestos removal is complete, special precautions
must be taken during cleanup because careless dusting,
sweeping, or vacuuming can spew fibers into the air.
All surfaces exposed to asbestos dust should be cleaned
at least twice with a wet mop and sponge. Sponges and
mops should be discarded or, at the very least, flushed
vigorously with running water after they are used. A
vacuum cleaner equipped with special filters designed
to capture asbestos fibers is a must; otherwise, most of
the fibers will pass through the vacuum cleaner bag
and be spewed back into the air.

• When cleanup is complete, removed asbestos products
and the plastic sheeting on the floor should be placed
in double, heavy-duty plastic garbage bags. Separate
the asbestos from the rest of the household trash and
call your local health department for disposal instructions.

FORMALDEHYDE

Formaldehyde, first synthesized in 1859, is an essential
chemical building block of textiles, pesticides, disinfectants,
wooden building materials, plastics, cosmetics, and numerous
other modern products. It is used to produce new chemicals

and to bind dissimilar compounds together to form new materials. Formaldehyde achieved fame back in 1909 when it was used in a chemical reaction that created the first entirely synthetic plastic material. At the time, it was touted as a miracle of the industrial age, and seers correctly predicted its widespread use in coming years.

Today, formaldehyde is used just about everywhere. Some 6.7 billion pounds of the colorless gas were produced in the United States in 1989, according to the *Chemical Marketing Reporter*. The forest products industry alone uses more than 500,000 tons of urea-formaldehyde resins each year to manufacture pressed wood products, which include:

- Particleboard, used as subflooring and shelving, and in cabinetry and furniture.
- Hardwood plywood paneling, used in decorative wall coverings, cabinets, and furniture.
- Medium-density fiberboard, used in cabinets and furniture.
- Softwood plywood, used in exterior construction.

Paper products, such as newsprint, waxed papers, and grocery bags, also contain formaldehyde, as do these common household products:

- Carpets, draperies, furniture fabrics, and permanent-press clothes, which are treated to resist mold and fire, to prevent shrinkage, and to make them crush-proof. The textile industry also uses formaldehyde to create new synthetic fibers and to act as a dye.
- Paints, shellacs, waxes, polishes, oils, and other coating materials, in which formaldehyde is used as a preservative. Even ferns and flowers are treated with a formaldehyde-based product to make them less perishable. The gas is also present in photography darkroom chemicals.
- Glues and adhesives, which use formaldehyde because of its excellent bonding characteristics and low cost.

- Molded plastics, which are used in hardware, plumbing fixtures, and automobiles. Gears, pulleys, pipes, zippers, combs, and bottles also contain formaldehyde.
- Insecticides, fumigants, disinfectants, deodorants, germicidal soaps, and embalming fluid, which use form-aldehyde to kill bacteria, fungi, molds, and yeasts.
- Cosmetics, including shampoos, nail hardeners, mouth-washes, and antiperspirants. Household cleaning products.

Small quantities of formaldehyde are also an end product of combustion and can be spewed into the air from cigarette smoke, and the burning of gas, wood, coal, oil, or kerosene. In congested urban areas, traces of formaldehyde can infil-trate a home, but this is rarely a significant source of the gas.

The UFFI Story

The most notorious source of formaldehyde comes from a material used to insulate nearly a half-million homes during the 1970s. Pumping urea-formaldehyde foam insulation (UFFI) into the walls was intended as an energy conservation measure, but its use sparked a barrage of health complaints, mostly relating to eye, nose, and throat irritations and skin rashes. Hundreds of families were actually forced to abandon their homes because the concentration of formaldehyde gas caused more severe symptoms, including nosebleeds, severe dizziness, and vomiting. In late 1979, the Chemical Industry Institute of Toxicology reported that the chemical caused cancer in rats. As a result of further studies and a public outcry, the Consumer Product Safety Commission issued a ban against UFFI in 1982.

But the story did not end there. The Formaldehyde Insti-tute, a trade association, challenged the ruling in federal court. The ban was overturned within nine months. While the court disputed the CPSC's claim that formaldehyde was carcinogenic, the surrounding publicity discouraged consum-ers and manufacturers alike from using the once-popular insulation. Although UFFI poses little threat if it is correctly mixed and applied in warm, dry weather, the product is rarely used today. But in the half-million houses and mobile homes where UFFI was added, improper installation still continues to cause problems.

What Are the Health Hazards?

Formaldehyde contaminates indoor spaces through a process called *outgassing*, a form of evaporation in which chemically unstable molecules are released into the air. The majority of formaldehyde in susceptible products evaporates quickly, but wood products that are glued together with urea-formaldehyde resins—notably, particleboard subflooring, paneling, cabinetry, furniture, medium-density fiberboard, and hardwood plywood paneling—pose a greater problem. The chemically unstable glue emits formaldehyde gas intensely during the first six months of a product's life and at reduced levels for as long as five years. Low-level outgassing continues indefinitely, particularly when indoor temperature and relative humidity levels are high.

The disquieting health effects of formaldehyde were first observed by the residents of mobile homes, which typically contain lots of particleboard and plywood paneling. Despite its popularity, formaldehyde is an irritant of the upper respiratory tract, and health effects typically mimic those of a cold. Symptoms include coughing, runny nose, sore throat, fatigue, and eye and sinus irritations. Skin rashes, dizziness, nausea, vomiting, and nosebleeds also have been reported. A number of studies have linked high levels of residential formaldehyde exposure with menstrual disorders; formaldehyde also has been blamed for chronic headaches and periodic memory lapses. Several years after court battles were waged over the UFFI ban, formaldehyde was labeled "a probable human carcinogen" by the Environmental Protection Agency; research continues in this disturbing area.

Individual sensitivity to formaldehyde varies quite a bit.

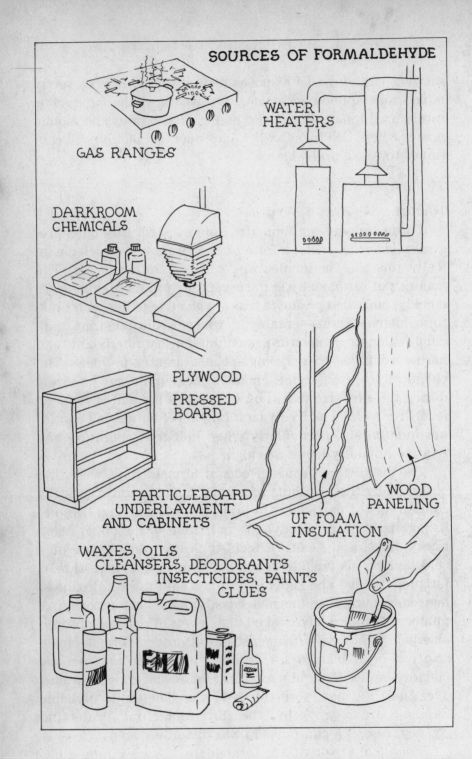

SOURCES OF FORMALDEHYDE

GAS RANGES

WATER HEATERS

DARKROOM CHEMICALS

PLYWOOD

PRESSED BOARD

PARTICLEBOARD UNDERLAYMENT AND CABINETS

UF FOAM INSULATION

WOOD PANELING

WAXES, OILS CLEANSERS, DEODORANTS INSECTICIDES, PAINTS GLUES

Some 10 to 20 percent of the population is highly sensitive to the gas and suffers ill effects even at low doses. Many people also react adversely to formaldehyde after being exposed to it over a long period of time. Asthmatics, young children, and others particularly susceptible to respiratory irritations are most likely to suffer adverse health effects.

Formaldehyde Concentrations
parts per million (ppm)*

2.00 ppm   Occupational Safety and Health Administration maximum standard for workplace exposure for a period not in excess of fifteen minutes.

1.00 ppm   Occupational Safety and Health Administration standard for workplace exposure, averaged over an eight-hour period.

0.5   ppm   Can cause burning of the eyes and irritation of the upper respiratory tract.

0.4   ppm   Formaldehyde emissions standard set by the U.S. Department of Housing and Urban Development for mobile homes.

0.25 ppm   Concentration level not irritating to most healthy adults, per the National Academy of Sciences.

0.10 ppm   Recommended maximum level of continual indoor exposure, per the American Society of Heating, Refrigeration and Air-conditioning Engineers.

*Formaldehyde is measured in parts per million (ppm). A measurement of 1 ppm indicates that one unit of formaldehyde is contained in one million units of air.

Testing for Formaldehyde

An easy-to-use monitor allows you to test the air in your home for the presence of formaldehyde. The monitor consists of a glass vial with a chemically treated filter on one end that is designed to capture airborne formaldehyde at a constant rate. The vial is left open on a countertop or table for the time period specified by a laboratory, generally about one week. Then, the vial is capped and returned to the lab so that the formaldehyde concentration can be measured. Formaldehyde monitors cost between $25 and $50, including the laboratory analysis.

Eliminating Formaldehyde

The best way to avoid exposure is to avoid products that contain formaldehyde, especially when remodeling or building a new home. Considering the ubiquitous uses for the product, that's admittedly no easy feat, but healthier alternatives do exist—solid-wood products are generally safer than glued wood, older furniture is less likely to emit fumes than new, and foam insulation can be replaced by fiberglass batting.

Fortunately, most formaldehyde outgasses during the first few weeks of a product's life. Within two to three years, formaldehyde emissions generally drop to half what they were when the product was new. Increasing the ventilation in your home and making a special effort to keep humidity levels low after a new purchase helps reduce the most toxic exposures. Here are some other ways to avoid formaldehyde:

• Find out how much of the noxious gas is contained in the item you are considering purchasing. The manufacturer should be able to supply this information, which can help you choose between competing products.
• Don't buy particleboard or pressed-wood products that use urea-formaldehyde glue. Plywood products graded for exterior use contain glue that emits little or no

formaldehyde. Specify that your cabinets be constructed of exterior plywood with solid-lumber fronts. This costs a little more, but the trade-off for sturdier and emission-free materials is a reasonable one.

- Paint over hardwood paneling or particleboard cabinets with a water-based sealant or polyurethane varnish to reduce formaldehyde emissions. Unless you are willing to dismantle the cabinets or take down the paneling, you won't be able to treat the whole product, but just painting easily accessible surfaces significantly reduces outgassing. Sealant needs to be reapplied every few years.

- Unless you are unusually sensitive or are planning a major remodeling project at the same time, it is generally impractical to remove urea-formaldehyde foam insulation. Walls must first be stripped down to the studs before the insulation can be cut and scraped out; afterwards, the wallboard and trim may have to be completely replaced. A better solution is to keep humidity levels low if UFFI is present, because the resins outgas more rapidly in humid conditions. In addition, any products containing UFFI resins should be dried as soon as possible if they become soaked. Finally, cracks on the indoor side of UFFI-filled exterior walls should be repaired and the walls painted with a vapor-barrier paint.

VOLATILE ORGANIC COMPOUNDS

Volatile organic compounds (VOCs) is the collective name given to the carbon-based gaseous contaminants emitted from a wide range of common household products. Typically, VOCs are found indoors at between two and five times the outdoor concentration, even in heavily industrialized areas. In one study that measured VOCs when paint stripper was used indoors, that figure soared one thousand times higher.

Both formaldehyde and some combustion by-products,

discussed in the next chapter, are VOCs, but there are hundreds of others, many with tongue-twisting names. Many VOCs are distilled from petroleum products, while others are synthetics produced by chemical reaction. Most products used in simple home repairs—from paint strippers and adhesive removers to paints and shellacs—emit some type of toxic fumes. Art materials are another often overlooked and potentially very hazardous source of VOCs. Among the chemical contaminants and the common household products in which VOCs are found:

- Solvents, which are liquids with the capacity to dissolve other substances, are used in lacquers, adhesives, waxes, cleaning agents, cosmetics, paints and paint removers, leather finishes, and inks. Common solvents include toluene, benzene, xylene, methyl cellosolve, ethyl cellosolve, methyl ethyl ketone, 1,1,1-trichloroethane (TCA), and trichloroethylene (TCE).
- Phenols, contained in household disinfectants, antiseptics, perfumes, mouthwashes, polishes, waxes, glues, and, ironically, air fresheners. They are also a byproduct of combustion. Phenols include biphenyl, phenolics, and the preservative pentachlorophenol (PCP).
- Aerosol sprays, which are propelled by propane, butane, and nitrous oxide gases. The American Lung Association says that some forty-five aerosol products can be found in a typical home.
- Permanent-press fabrics, polyesters, and other synthetic materials, which release chemical fumes into the air as they age. Drapes and furniture also contain VOCs, and the dry-cleaning process drenches fabrics in perchloroethylene, tetrachloroethylene, and other hazardous chemicals.
- Pesticides, estimated to be found in nine out of ten American households. The EPA believes as much as 90 percent of the general public's exposure to pesticides

occurs indoors. They can be carried in from the out-doors and are also used in disinfectants, pet collars, and plant food, and to combat infestations of ants, cockroaches, termites, and other insects. Pesticides can remain chemically active for years. Traces of chlordane, aldrin, dieldrin, and heptachlor, once common ingredients of termiticides, are found in the air inside many homes even today, although all have been banned for several years. These insecticides are extremely toxic—all are suspected of causing cancer and other serious diseases in humans.

• Electrical equipment and some plastics, which contain the notorious polychlorinated biphenyls (PCBs). PCBs are actually a group of 200 fire-resistant compounds that do not readily break down or disperse. If they are improperly discarded, they can seep into the ground-water, be transported through the air as vapor, or attach themselves to dust particles. When they are inhaled or absorbed through the skin, PCBs accumulate in the body's fatty tissue.

What Are the Health Hazards?

Exposure to individual VOCs are associated with a range of health hazards, from eye irritations and upper respiratory tract infections to metabolic disorders. Paint fumes frequently cause headaches, nausea, and respiratory problems in sensitive individuals and eventually lead to liver and kidney disorders. Some organic chemicals have even been identified as potential carcinogens in occupational and animal toxicity studies. Among the VOCs with known or suspected cancer-causing properties are benzene, TCE, TCA, methylene chloride, perchloroethylene, and PCBs.

The adhesives used when wall-to-wall carpeting is installed are a common source of complaints—the Consumer Product Safety Commission reports that one woman became nauseous after visiting a home in which carpeting had been installed and another developed a body rash and had breathing difficulties. Pesticide chemicals also pose clear health risks. In one instance, a jury awarded $400,000 to a Georgia family whose members suffered from headaches, blurry vision, and a variety of other flulike symptoms after a termiticide was inadvertently sprayed on a deck outside the house and in the hollow cinder blocks of the foundation.

The Art Hazards Information Center in New York says the health problems associated with exposure to certain art materials probably includes skin irritations, respiratory problems, mood swings, fatigue, headaches, mercury poisoning, an increased risk of miscarriage, and cancer. The center has documented numerous cases of persons suffering dire consequences from the use of art materials, including a jewelry maker with cadmium poisoning, a batik artist who cannot stop coughing, and a teacher who suffered brain damage after using solvents and chemicals in the silk-screening process.

Workplace exposures and a famous accident in Japan, in which a number of people ate rice oil contaminated with PCBs, have told us quite a bit about the health effects of such incidents. Symptoms associated with acute, short-term exposure to PCBs include headache, fatigue, skin eruptions, nausea, digestive problems, liver dysfunction, and reproductive problems. With long-term exposure, PCBs are likely human carcinogens and can cause low birth weight.

Unfortunately, the majority of volatile organic compounds in household and industrial use today have not received thorough scientific scrutiny. Complete information about associated health risks is simply unavailable. It is likely, however, that low-level exposure to a combination of VOCs over a long period of time may pose cumulative hazards that are more alarming than acute, short-term exposure to a single compound. Research into VOCs is one of the most important avenues of pollution-related scientific investigation being pursued today.

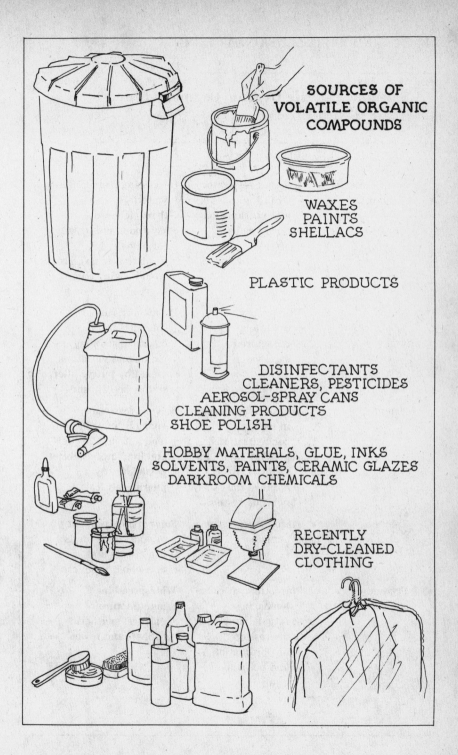

SOURCES OF
VOLATILE ORGANIC
COMPOUNDS

WAXES
PAINTS
SHELLACS

PLASTIC PRODUCTS

DISINFECTANTS
CLEANERS, PESTICIDES
AEROSOL-SPRAY CANS
CLEANING PRODUCTS
SHOE POLISH

HOBBY MATERIALS, GLUE, INKS
SOLVENTS, PAINTS, CERAMIC GLAZES
DARKROOM CHEMICALS

RECENTLY
DRY-CLEANED
CLOTHING

Selected Volatile Organic Compounds and Their Health Effects

Compound	Health Effects	Sources and Uses
Formaldehyde and other aldehydes	Eye and respiratory irritation; possibly more serious long-term health effects	Outgassing from building materials (particleboard, plywood, and urea-formaldehyde insulation foam); also from cooking and smoking
Benzene	Respiratory irritation; recognized carcinogen	Plastic and rubber solvents; from cigarette smoking; in paints and varnishes, including putty, filler, stains, and finishes
Xylene	Narcotic; irritating; in high concentrations, possibly injurious to heart, liver, kidney, and nervous system	Solvent for resins, enamels, etc.; in non-lead automobile fuels and in manufacture of pesticides, dyes, pharmaceuticals
Toluene	Narcotic; may cause anemia	Solvents; by-product of organic compounds used in several household products
Styrene	Narcotic; can cause headache, fatigue, stupor, depression, incoordination, and possible eye injury	Widespread in manufacture of plastics, synthetic rubber, and resins

Compound	Health Effects	Sources and Uses
Trichloroethane	Subject of OSHA carcinogenesis inquiry	Aerosol propellant, pesticide, cleaning solvent
Trichloroethylene	Animal carcinogen; subject of OSHA carcinogenesis inquiry	Oil and wax solvents, cleaning compounds, vapor degreasing products, dry-cleaning operations; also as an anesthetic
Ethyl benzene	Severe irritation to eyes and respiratory system	Solvents; in styrene-related products
Chloro benzenes	Strong narcotic; possible lung, liver, and kidney damage	In production of paint, varnish, pesticides, and various organic solvents
Polychlorinated biphenyls (PCBs)	Suspected carcinogens	In various electrical components; in waste oil supplies, and in plastic and paper products in which PCBs are used as plasticizers
Pesticides	Suspected carcinogens	Insect control

SOURCE: C. D. Hollowell and R. R. Miksch, *Sources and Concentrations of Organic Compounds in Indoor Environments*, Lawrence Berkeley Laboratory Report LBL-13195 (July 1981). Reprinted courtesy of Lawrence Berkeley Laboratory.

Testing for Volatile Organic Compounds

Because there are literally thousands of volatile organic compounds in common use today, it is both impractical and meaningless to test the indoor air for the presence of each one. A good rule of thumb instead is to use as many chemical-free products as possible and to eliminate the source of VOCs wherever you can.

Eliminating Volatile Organic Compounds

Wearing natural fabrics, installing carpeting and drapery with a minimum of chemical additives and dyes, and purchasing toxic-free cleaning products are sensible and practical safeguards against excess chemical exposure. These days, that's easier than ever, because a variety of manufacturers now specialize in supplying nontoxic products for construction and ordinary household chores.

Here are the three other broad guidelines for reducing the hazards of contaminating volatile organic compounds:

- First, read the fine print on product labels. Find out what's in a product and what precautions are recommended by the manufacturer for its proper use. Be sure to follow the directions to the letter.
- Second, provide adequate ventilation when using VOC-rich products. Open some windows, turn on an exhaust fan, and, whenever possible, take hobby or cleaning projects outside. See Chapter 5 for more on this subject.
- Third, store paint, fuel, and pesticides in a garage or shed, or at least in a well-ventilated part of your house or apartment. Even tightly sealed cans allow active ingredients to leak out, so get in the habit of buying only as much as you need—that way, there will be no leftovers to worry about.

HOUSEHOLD CLEANERS: Unfortunately, products designed to take the strain out of housework generally enlist toxic chemical helpers to do the job. You can improve indoor air quality without sacrificing cleanliness by using the least-toxic product available and by following these guidelines:

- Avoid chlorine bleach, a component of most household cleansers. Bleach releases chlorine gas, which is an irritant to the nose and eyes. Products containing chlorine should never be mixed with ammonia, vinegar, or toilet bowl cleaner—the combination can be deadly. One teaspoon of borax and a dash of vinegar mixed in a quart of water is an effective substitute for commercial chlorine- and ammonia-based cleansers.
- Don't use oven cleaners, which are rich in lye and other hazardous chemicals. Wiping the oven out after every use helps it stay clean, and keeping a cookie sheet or aluminum foil in the bottom of the oven is a good way to catch spills. When the oven does collect dirt and grease, it can be cleaned with a homemade solution of water and baking soda. Spread the mixture, wait for it to dry, then wipe it off with a damp cloth.
- Air fresheners make your home smell better by anesthetizing your nose, not by removing the odor-causing substance. Rather than use toxic chemicals in a misplaced attempt to purify the air, you can usually keep the house smelling fresh just by opening a window. Placing an open dish of heated vinegar in the kitchen or bathroom helps clear the air, and an open box of baking soda inside the refrigerator will absorb many food odors. A bouquet of fresh flowers and flowering plants are other natural deodorizers.
- Avoid aerosol sprays. While convenient, the propellants used to force hair spray, deodorant, oven cleaner, air freshener, and myriad other products out of the can are toxic.
- Don't buy shoe polish that contains nitrobenzene, trichloroethylene, or methylene chloride, all potential carcinogens. Avoid any product that doesn't list its contents on the label.

CONSTRUCTION AND HOBBY MATERIALS: Good ventilation can minimize many of the disquieting hazards of popular home repair and art and hobby materials. The Center for Safety in the Arts can provide numerous other specific suggestions for the safe use of such materials. Here are some other ways to protect yourself:

- Substitute latex for oil-based paints, which require toxic paint thinner. Some people also prefer to avoid latex paints because they contain toxic-emitting acrylics and fungicides. While all-natural paints pigmented with plant oils or minerals are available, they are costly, not as durable as synthetics, and impractical for all but the most committed purist. A more reasonable compromise is to stick with latex paints while providing as much outdoor air as possible for a day or two after painting to clear away the fumes.
- Try not to use paint stripper indoors, because it emits toxic fumes, including methylene chloride. If you must remove paint, provide as much ventilation as possible and wear a respirator designed to intercept volatile chemicals.
- If the exposed beams inside your home are emitting a strong chemical smell, they have probably been treated with a preservative, such as pentachlorophenol or creosote, to protect them from bug infestation and rot. Stop the outgassing by sealing the beams with at least two coats of polyurethane varnish.
- Learn what's in the art supplies you buy. Seek out materials with the Certified Label (CL) seal from the Arts and Crafts Materials Institute. The label will include information written by a toxicologist on that particular product's hazards; any warnings should be taken seriously. You should also request a material safety data sheet (MSDS), which manufacturers of hazardous products are required to provide under the Occupational Safety and Health Administration's Hazards Communications Standard.
- Substitute safer products for hazardous ones whenever possible. Water-based paints are better than oil-based ones, solvent-rich felt tip markers should be avoided,

and poster paints are preferable to leaded glazes. Avoid paint that comes in aerosol cans and use liquid products rather than products in a dry or powdered form.

- Don't eat food while working with art or hobby materials, because this increases the likelihood of ingesting or inhaling hazardous materials.
- Wear protective clothing, including gloves and a long-sleeved shirt, when working with solvents. Use safety goggles when grinding, sanding, or welding, and wear a face mask if you must work with powders, dusts, or fumes. Work outside whenever possible and remove clothing before leaving the work area.
- Ceramics projects are especially threatening to indoor air quality because extremely toxic chemicals are often used in glazes, the kilns used to fire pottery emit poisonous vapors, and clay dust can easily become airborne. Be sure to wear a dust mask when mixing glazes or hydrating powdered clay and work outside, or at least in a well-ventilated room, preferably one that is isolated from the rest of the house. Locate your kiln outdoors if possible.

CLOTHING: Winter woolens can be safely stored in a cedar chest, cedar-lined drawers, or boxes packed with cedar blocks, rather than mothballs, which contain paradichlorobenzene and other harmful chemicals. If you do use mothballs, pack your clothes away in an attic chest, an outdoor shed, a garage, or at least a distant closet. Be sure to air out your clothes thoroughly before wearing them or putting them back into the bedroom closet.

Find a dry cleaner who does not return your clothes to you with a strong chemical smell. It's a good idea to hang dry-cleaned clothes outdoors or in a well-ventilated room before putting them away.

PESTICIDES: Avoid the use of pesticides as much as possible. Keep a flyswatter handy and don't hesitate to use it. Bar entry to rodents by filling any cracks or holes in the walls with steel wool or by covering holes with metal screens. Traps, if you have the stomach for them, are also superior to chemical poisons. Keep a close eye on your houseplants and isolate any that become bug-infested. Bug repellent and indoor insecticides made from nontoxic components are now commercially available, or you can consult a book on organic gardening to learn how to make your own.

Termiticides are especially toxic. A better way to deter termites is to keep inviting wood scraps and firewood away from the house. Metal termite shields can be installed on the top of a building's foundation during new construction to prevent the pests from crawling into the structure's wood framework. All wood scraps should be removed before the trench excavated for the foundation is filled again.

Be careful when hiring a professional pest control company to rid your home of termites, cockroaches, or other persistent insects. Along with checking references and comparing prices, you should ask for a written control program that specifies what chemicals will be used and how they will be applied.

3
THE PERILS OF NATURE
Radon and Biological Agents

As if the pollution released from synthetic products were not alarming enough, Mother Nature also makes a contribution to indoor contamination. Two of the most common pollutants in the home actually originate outside, from natural sources. Radon gas, which cannot be seen, smelled, or tasted, seeps into the basement from soil and rocks. Fortunately, easy-to-run tests make radon easy to detect, and there are a variety of effective ways to eliminate the gas.

More immediately obvious is the discomfort caused by biological contaminants, including spores from mold and fungi, pollen from outdoor trees and plants, and disease-carrying organisms, such as bacteria, viruses, and parasites. Again, solutions to the problem are within the ready reach of most homeowners and renters.

Here's a closer look at radon and biological agents.

RADON

In a scene that evoked Meryl Streep's memorable performance in *Silkwood*, Stanley Watras, an engineer at the Limerick nuclear power plant in Sanatoga, Pennsylvania, repeatedly triggered the facility's radiation monitor as he headed home from work. Since there was not yet fuel in the reactor, power plant officials were understandably bewildered by the emergency signal—until the morning Watras triggered the alarm as he entered the building. That's when everyone realized Watras was actually carrying radiation *into* his workplace. Subsequent tests revealed radon levels in his home so high that the health risk was estimated to be the equivalent of smoking more than 100 packs of cigarettes every day.

Stanley Watras's story is extreme, but concern about the colorless, tasteless, and odorless gas has escalated over the past few years. Radon is a naturally occurring gas released by a chain of radioactive decay that is as old as the Earth itself. Uranium, a ubiquitous component of the Earth's crust, breaks down into radium, which in turn releases radon as its first decay product. Radon gas is inert, meaning that it does not react with other chemicals, but it, too, decays, emitting submicroscopic particles known as radon daughters.

Radon and radon daughters can penetrate a home when uranium is present in nearby soil and rock. Granite, shale, and phosphate bedrock, as well as soils and gravel derived from these sources, are most likely to contain uranium and its decay products. Certain geological formations—such as the

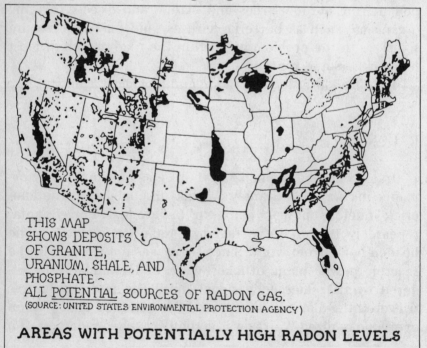

THIS MAP
SHOWS DEPOSITS
OF GRANITE,
URANIUM, SHALE, AND
PHOSPHATE –
ALL POTENTIAL SOURCES OF RADON GAS.
(SOURCE: UNITED STATES ENVIRONMENTAL PROTECTION AGENCY)

AREAS WITH POTENTIALLY HIGH RADON LEVELS

Reading Prong, which cuts a broad swath across New York, New Jersey, and Pennsylvania—are especially rich in uranium deposits. By contrast, regions where dark volcanic rocks are prevalent seldom have a radon problem.

Radon gas passes undetected through cracks in a building foundation, joints in concrete slabs, loose-fitting gas and water pipes, drains, and sumps. Well water is a less-publicized source: The EPA estimates that as much as half the radon found inside homes in the Northeast has evaporated from household water. Interior construction materials, such as gypsum wallboard and concrete, even stoneware pottery, can also emit small amounts of radon if the components from which they are made contain traces of uranium.

A seventeen-state, 20,000-home EPA survey has uncovered unacceptably high radon levels across the country—more than 25 percent of tested homes exceeded the concentration at which corrective action is recommended. Because radon tends to concentrate in a basement or the lower floors of a

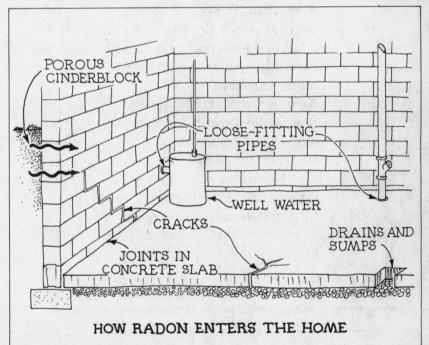

HOW RADON ENTERS THE HOME

building, it rarely poses a problem to apartment dwellers, but as many as eight million houses, located in every state, are likely to contain unsafe levels of radon. While local public health officials know whether radon is common in a particular region, concentrations are highly unpredictable. In fact, measurements taken in neighboring houses can differ markedly. The only accurate way to know whether a home is contaminated with radon is to test for it. In the fall of 1988, the Environmental Protection Agency and the U.S. Surgeon General issued a widely publicized health advisory urging that all homes be tested for the presence of radon. Shortly afterward, a similar warning was issued for the nation's schools.

Radon Concentrations
picocuries per liter (pCi/L)*

16 pCi/L   Maximum allowable radon exposure for miners, per U.S. Mines Safety and Health Administration regulations.

8 pCi/L   Level at which the National Council on Radiation, Protection and Measurement advises the general population to reduce radon exposure.

5 pCi/L   Average wintertime level at which the Bonneville Power Administration advises individuals undertaking energy conservation measures to reduce radon exposure.

4 pCi/L   The Environmental Protection Agency's target annual average concentration level for the general population.

1 pCi/L   Average level of radon found in U.S. homes.

*Radon concentration is measured in picocuries per liter. A picocurie is one-trillionth of a curie, a standard unit of radiation. One pCi/L represents the decay of 2.2 atoms of radon per liter of air per minute.

What Are the Health Hazards?

Concern about the dangers of radon originated with uranium miners, who are exposed to a hundred times the level typically found indoors and whose lung cancer rates are significantly higher than those of the general population. The catastrophic effects of high-dose radiation exposure has also been studied among atomic bomb survivors, and the long-term consequences are genuinely horrifying. The general population, of course, is exposed to comparatively tiny doses

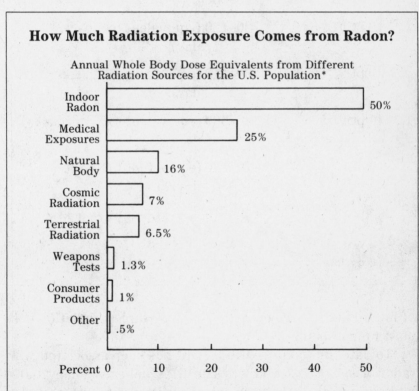

How Much Radiation Exposure Comes from Radon?

Annual Whole Body Dose Equivalents from Different Radiation Sources for the U.S. Population*

Source	Percent
Indoor Radon	50%
Medical Exposures	25%
Natural Body	16%
Cosmic Radiation	7%
Terrestrial Radiation	6.5%
Weapons Tests	1.3%
Consumer Products	1%
Other	.5%

Percent 0   10   20   30   40   50

*Percentages exceed 100 percent due to rounding.

SOURCE: "Indoor Air Pollutant—Radon." Bodanski, Jackson, and Geraci. Courtesy of Washington Energy Extension Service, 914 East Jefferson, #300, Seattle, Wash. 98122. (206) 296-5640.

Lung Cancer Risks: How Radon Compares with Smoking

Lifetime Exposure picocuries per liter (pCi/L)	Estimated Radon Deaths/1,000 people exposed
1 pCi/L	3–13
2 pCi/L	7–30
4 pCi/L	13–50
10 pCi/L	30–120 (equivalent to 1 pack a day)
20 pCi/L	60–210 (equivalent to 2 packs a day)
40 pCi/L	120–380 (equivalent to 2½ packs a day)
100 pCi/L	270–630 (equivalent to 3 packs a day)
200 pCi/L	440–770 (equivalent to 4 packs a day)

SOURCE: "Radon Detectors," *Consumer Reports*, July 1987, pp. 440-43.

of radon, but this exposure is the single largest radiation dose most human beings receive.

To date, only one health hazard has been associated with radon gas, but it's a killer: The EPA believes some 20,000 lung cancer deaths a year are caused by exposure to radon decay products, making it the largest source of the agonizing disease after cigarette smoking. Radon can attach itself to dust particles, which are then inhaled, or the gas itself can be inhaled directly into the lungs. In either case, the process of decay continues in the lung tissue, unleashing damaging radiation.

A number of agencies have promulgated guidelines for limiting radon exposure, but it is impossible to say just how dangerous long-term, low-level exposure really is. Until more conclusive data becomes available, however, experts agree that any radon pollution poses a genuine environmental threat and should be monitored closely.

Testing for Radon

Many thousands of Americans have already followed the Environmental Protection Agency's recommendation to test their homes for the presence of radon. Increasingly, people interested in buying a home are also insisting on radon test results first. Often a house purchase contract will include a clause making the seller responsible for bringing radon levels down to an agreed-upon concentration level before the sale is finalized. Not surprisingly, a cottage industry of manufacturers who supply radon test equipment and evaluate the results has sprung up in the past few years.

Two types of easy-to-use radon detectors are available: activated-charcoal detectors and alpha-track devices. In-

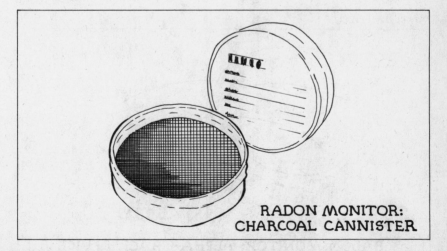

RADON MONITOR:
CHARCOAL CANNISTER

structions are included with the equipment, but no special expertise is required. *Charcoal detectors*, which absorb radon gas, are placed in a cool, dry spot in the basement for no more than a week, then sealed and sent to a laboratory for analysis. The canisters, which cost from $10 to $25 apiece (generally, at least two are necessary to get an accurate reading), are most useful for obtaining a fast indication of the extent of a problem.

Alpha-track devices are generally recommended for more accurate, long-term results and as a follow-up to a charcoal detector measurement. Alpha particles created during the process of radon decay strike a strip of special plastic material on the device, leaving microscopic track marks that can be counted in a laboratory. Alpha-track devices cost only a few dollars more than charcoal canisters but take a minimum of four weeks to obtain results.

To obtain the most accurate test results, either radon detector should be placed in the lowest room of the house, usually the basement. Beginning twelve hours before the testing period and continuing throughout the test, doors and windows should be kept closed as much as possible to prevent dilution and to keep radon levels relatively consistent. Wind

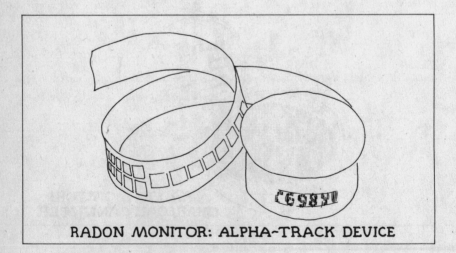

RADON MONITOR: ALPHA-TRACK DEVICE

and high humidity can distort results, so it is best to avoid testing during these weather conditions. Because of the high humidity levels, a radon detector should not be used in the kitchen or bathroom.

Laboratory results will be sent back to you a few days after your detector is received. Results are reported in picocuries per liter (pCi/L). The EPA has issued the following guidelines for determining the urgency of implementing radon reduction techniques:

- If the screening measurement is greater than 200 pCi/L, you have a serious radon problem that should be corrected as quickly as possible. In addition to follow-up measures to confirm the accuracy of the first result, prompt mitigation action is crucial.
- Measurements between 20 pCi/L and 200 pCi/L are significantly above average for residences. If your results fall within this range, radon detectors should be exposed for no longer than three months in follow-up testing. Meanwhile, mitigation measures should be implemented.
- If the screening measurement falls between 4 pCi/L and 20 pCi/L, follow-up measurements are advisable but the urgency is reduced. Detectors should be exposed for a full year, or for four one-week periods during each of the four seasons.
- Measurements below 4 pCi/L are about average for most residential structures. This is considered a relatively low concentration level, and follow-up measurements are generally not required.

If initial testing shows high levels of radon concentration, follow-up measurements should be taken on every floor, preferably in the most frequently used rooms, such as bedrooms. Once you have taken measures to eliminate radon, you'll want to use alpha-track detectors again to be certain that the problem has been eliminated.

Eliminating Radon

The good news about radon is that just about any infiltration problem is correctable. In the community of Clinton, New Jersey, for example, 105 houses were tested and *all* were found to have levels that exceeded EPA guidelines. This was the highest density of high-radon homes ever found, yet every affected homeowner was able to take steps that brought contamination down to an acceptable range.

Mitigation techniques fall into two broad categories: controlling radon at the source so that it doesn't enter your home or diluting it with fresh air once it gets inside. Until radon levels are reduced, try to minimize the amount of time you spend in the basement. As an interim measure, you can also bar radon entry into your living space by installing weather stripping on the door separating the first floor from the basement and by stapling a vapor barrier to the basement ceiling.

CAVEAT EMPTOR: Unless you are highly skilled in home renovations, you probably will need professional help to relieve a severe radon problem. Unfortunately, recent media attention has generated enough public concern to spawn some unscrupulous practices—we've heard stories about "black boxes," fluorescent lights, and other devices being peddled with the promise that they will eliminate radon from the home. Taking the time to understand the basic principles of radon mitigation is the best way to avoid a scam.

Here are some ways to reduce radon levels in your home:

SEAL BASEMENT CRACKS: To prevent the entry of radon through the building foundation, a homeowner should first take steps to seal cracks and openings in the basement walls and floors through which the gas can penetrate. This is a relatively inexpensive technique, but it rarely solves the whole problem because radon can often find passageways that even the most fastidious contractor has overlooked.

Cracks are typically found near drains, utility pipes, ventilation ducts, and at the joint where the floor meets the

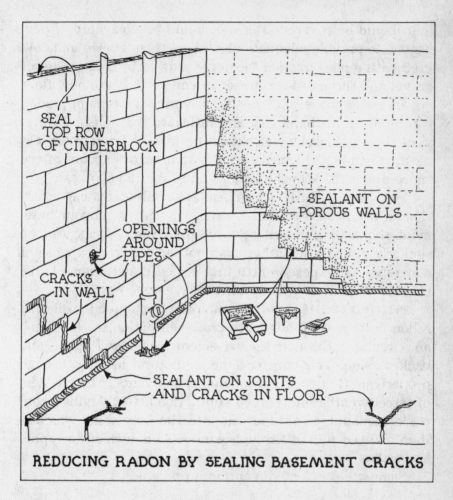

SEAL TOP ROW OF CINDERBLOCK

SEALANT ON POROUS WALLS

OPENINGS AROUND PIPES

CRACKS IN WALL

SEALANT ON JOINTS AND CRACKS IN FLOOR

REDUCING RADON BY SEALING BASEMENT CRACKS

walls. An epoxy sealant or an acrylic caulk to which synthetic rubber such as silicone has been added is an effective barrier against radon. Porous basement walls can also be coated with waterproof paint, cement plaster, or epoxy to block radon entry. Hollow or porous concrete blocks, which are frequently part of a building foundation, can be plugged with concrete, mortar, urethane foam, or an impermeable sealant.

COVER EXPOSED EARTH: Exposed earth in the basement or crawl space is frequently a major source of radon penetration and should be covered. The soil should be excavated, if necessary, to provide adequate clearance, then leveled and covered with a plastic vapor barrier, followed by four inches of gravel and three to four inches of concrete. If the new floor covers an air space, such as that around a sump pump, radon can build up in the cavity and infiltrate the house. To prevent this, a small blower should be installed wherever it is most convenient. Ideally, the pipe that carries air out of the space under the slab should extend to roof level.

You can also construct an insulated wall with a vapor barrier on the heated side to isolate any portion of your basement that is unfinished or unused. A crawl space can be similarly sealed off. Rather than bother with the expense of concrete, the exposed earth in a sealed crawl space can be covered with heavy plastic sheeting.

PROVIDE VENTILATION: The simplest technique for diluting radon is to provide adequate cross-ventilation so that fresh air circulates through the basement and crawl space and back outside. This can be done by natural means, through properly positioned windows, doors, and vents or by a system of forced ventilation. Forced ventilation actually pulls a controlled amount of outdoor air into the basement, which is then allowed to exit through windows on adjacent or opposite walls.

Some other effective ventilation techniques:

- Heat-Recovery Ventilation: The air-to-air heat exchangers discussed in some depth in Chapter 3 are an energy-saving way to exhaust radon-contaminated basement air and replace it with preheated outdoor air. A wall-mounted heat exchanger installed in a basement window works best where radon concentrations are relatively low. In homes with severe radon problems, a larger-capacity floor-mounted system is more appropriate.
- Sub-Slab Ventilation: If your basement floor consists of a concrete slab over gravel, sub-slab ventilation can

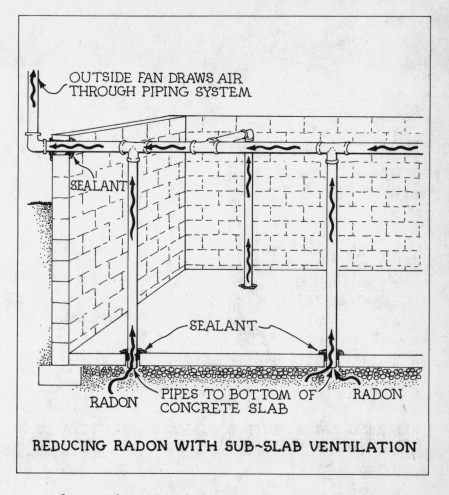

REDUCING RADON WITH SUB-SLAB VENTILATION

force radon-tainted air away from the house. Holes are first cut through the basement floor, and vertical pipes are installed with one end flush against the bottom of the concrete slab and sealed in place with rubberized caulk. The network of pipes is connected and routed outdoors above the top of the foundation or through upstairs walls and out the roof. A blower is installed near the outdoor termination of the piping system to suck air continually from under the slab.

• Block-Wall Ventilation: Venting the hollow space within the concrete blocks used in some foundations is

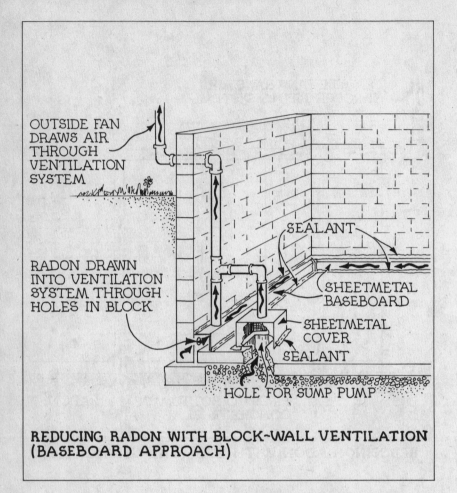

OUTSIDE FAN DRAWS AIR THROUGH VENTILATION SYSTEM

RADON DRAWN INTO VENTILATION SYSTEM THROUGH HOLES IN BLOCK

SEALANT

SHEETMETAL BASEBOARD

SHEETMETAL COVER

SEALANT

HOLE FOR SUMP PUMP

REDUCING RADON WITH BLOCK-WALL VENTILATION (BASEBOARD APPROACH)

another way to mitigate radon problems. A series of exhaust pipes is installed through holes cut into the block wall, and an outside blower is used to pull the radon through the blocks, into the piping, and out of the house. In a variation of this technique, baseboard ducts are installed around the basement perimeter and holes are drilled to connect the ducts with the hollow interior of the concrete block. A blower again pulls radon away. Block-wall ventilation is only effective if the top of the foundation wall and any cracks in its surface are thoroughly sealed.

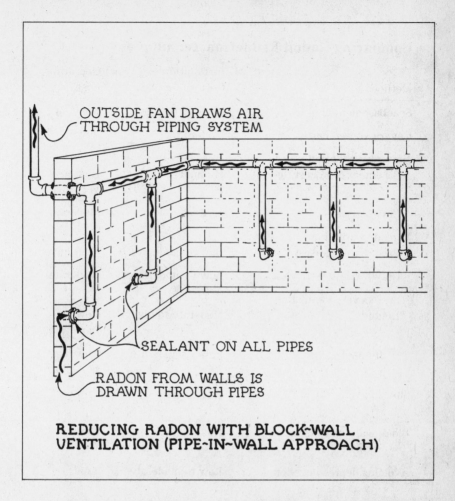

OUTSIDE FAN DRAWS AIR
THROUGH PIPING SYSTEM

SEALANT ON ALL PIPES

RADON FROM WALLS IS
DRAWN THROUGH PIPES

**REDUCING RADON WITH BLOCK-WALL
VENTILATION (PIPE-IN-WALL APPROACH)**

- Drain-Tile Suction: In many homes, a system of perforated plastic pipes or concrete drain tiles are positioned to drain water away from the foundation wall. The drain pipes are installed at the base of the foundation, usually all the way around the house, and the water that is collected drains into a sump. By attaching an exhaust fan to the drainage system at the point where it empties into the sump, radon can often be pulled from the soil before it infiltrates the basement or crawl space. Drain-tile suction can also be used where there is a basement floor drain connected to the perimeter

Comparing Radon Reduction Techniques

Method	Installation Cost	Operating Cost
Seal basement cracks	Minimal to high	Nominal
Cover exposed earth	Moderate to high	Low
Natural ventilation		
Basement or lowest floor	Minimal	High to very high
Crawl space	Minimal	Moderate
Forced ventilation		
Basement or lowest floor	Low to moderate	Very high
Crawl space	Low to moderate	Moderate
Heat-recovery ventilation		
Ducted	Moderate to high	Low to moderate
Wall-mounted	Low to moderate	Low to moderate
Sub-slab ventilation	High	Low
Block-wall ventilation	High	Low
Avoiding depressurization	Low to moderate	Low
House pressurization	Moderate to high	Moderate

*These represent the best reductions in radon levels that can be expected with a single method. Actual reductions may be considerably lower and can vary, depending on the particular characteristics of your house. Several methods may have to be combined to achieve acceptable results.

Maximum Possible Radon Reduction*	Comment
Site specific	Required to make most other methods work.
Site specific	Required to make most other methods work.
Up to 90 percent	Useful immediate step to reduce high radon levels.
Up to 90 percent	
Up to 90 percent	More controlled than natural ventilation.
Up to 90 percent	
50 to 75 percent	Air intake and exhaust must be equal. Radon reduction is less for houses with moderate to high air exchange rates.
No data available	
Up to 99 percent	Works best with good aggregate or highly permeable soil under slab.
Up to 99 percent	Applies to block-wall basements. Sub-slab suction may be needed to supplement.
Site specific	May be required to make other methods work. May see seasonal impact.
Up to 90 percent (limited data)	Most cost-effective when basement is tightly sealed.

*These represent the best reductions in radon levels that can be expected with a single method. Actual reductions may be considerably lower and can vary, depending on the particular characteristics of your house. Several methods may have to be combined to achieve acceptable results.

SOURCE: "Radon Reduction Methods: A Homeowner's Guide," Environmental Protection Agency, August 1986.

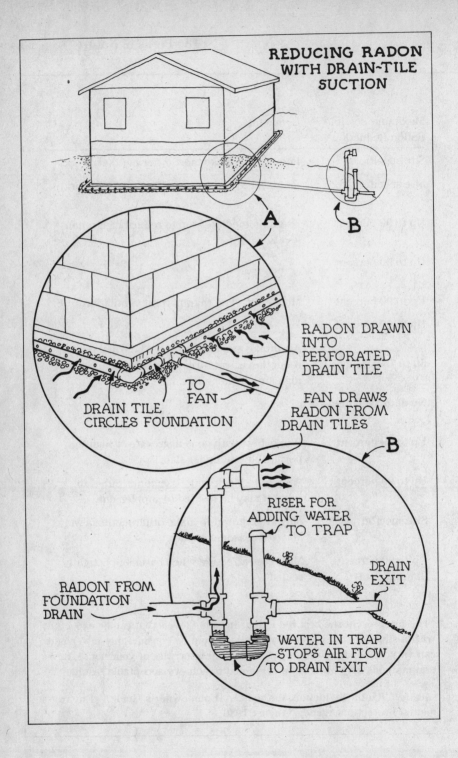

REDUCING RADON WITH DRAIN-TILE SUCTION

A

B

RADON DRAWN INTO PERFORATED DRAIN TILE

TO FAN

FAN DRAWS RADON FROM DRAIN TILES

DRAIN TILE CIRCLES FOUNDATION

B

RISER FOR ADDING WATER TO TRAP

DRAIN EXIT

RADON FROM FOUNDATION DRAIN

WATER IN TRAP STOPS AIR FLOW TO DRAIN EXIT

drainage system. However, this technique is only effective if there is a trap on the basement drain that is
kept full of water.

AVOID DEPRESSURIZATION: A number of household appliances and heating devices remove interior air, creating a
slight vacuum that can pull radon gas inside. Vented exhaust
fans and clothes dryers, as well as wood stoves, fireplaces,
and furnaces, which consume oxygen to support combustion,
are the usual culprits.

The least expensive way to avoid the depressurization
problem is to keep a window cracked slightly open near such
appliances. Providing the stove and fireplace with a source
of fresh air through a system of ducts or pipes is an energy-
efficient, although costly, way to eliminate the effects of
negative pressure. If possible, you can enclose the furnace in
a separate basement area and vent it to the outdoors.

A related technique for eliminating radon is to pressurize
the basement slightly by installing a fan in the upstairs floor
to push air down into the basement or crawl space.

BIOLOGICAL AGENTS

A host of microscopic organisms—including bacteria, viruses, fungi, molds, mildews, and mites—can multiply indoors and cause discomfort or illness. Airborne pollen, which
is actually a collection of spores from seed-bearing grasses,
flowers, and trees, also belongs on this list. People, pets, even
insects can pick up these biological agents outside and carry
them indoors, or they can be brought in with the air that
penetrates through doors, windows, vents, and cracks in the
building envelope. Dander and hair of people and pets are
other organic materials that contribute to indoor air pollution. Incredibly, the leading source of nutrition for household

microbes is the three grams of skin that flake off the average human body every day.

Once they establish an indoor foothold, microbes can flourish in even the cleanest of American homes. To thrive, they need food, moisture, and breeding grounds, generally finding them in areas where there are leaks or condensation. Windowsills, indoor walls beneath windows, bathrooms, carpet padding, the area behind baseboard trim, humidifiers, refrigerator drip pans, central air conditioning systems, heating ducts, and ice machines all provide a moist environment in which biological agents can thrive. These often-unseen microbes are most likely to multiply when relative indoor humidity levels are high.

In a tightly sealed house, a surprising amount of moisture can accumulate as a consequence of ordinary household activities. A family of four generates 12 pints of water every day simply because they breathe and sweat. Four people watching a television thriller can release more than a pint of moisture every hour just by breathing hard and sweating copiously. Another 12 pints of moisture can evaporate into the air daily while the family bathes, cooks, does the laundry, and washes the dishes. Additional moisture comes from appliances that use water, such as the washing machine or dishwasher, as well as damp basements, indoor saunas, leaks in the roof or the plumbing system, accidental spills, and houseplants.

Pets also carry biological agents indoors, and their saliva and urine readily attract microbial growth. Cat urine is a particularly common allergen. Even if it contains the latest disinfectants and odor-neutralizing chemicals, a cat's litter box can become a source of airborne bacteria and disagreeable odors.

What Are the Health Hazards?

Biological agents can be inhaled directly or can attach

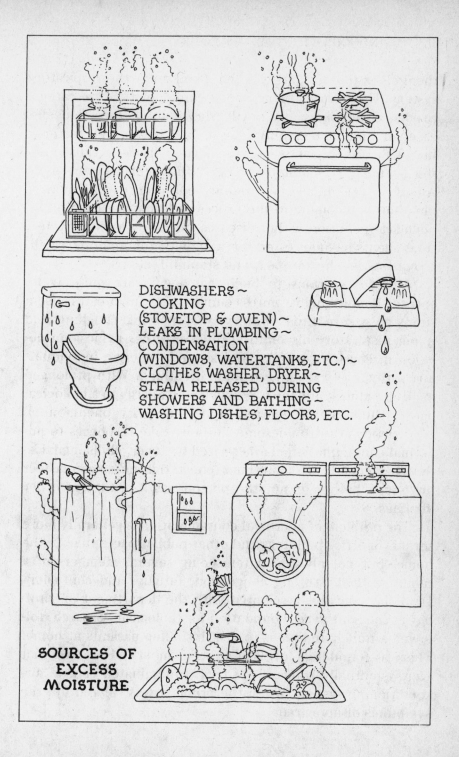

DISHWASHERS ~
COOKING
(STOVETOP & OVEN) ~
LEAKS IN PLUMBING ~
CONDENSATION
(WINDOWS, WATERTANKS, ETC.) ~
CLOTHES WASHER, DRYER ~
STEAM RELEASED DURING
SHOWERS AND BATHING ~
WASHING DISHES, FLOORS, ETC.

SOURCES OF
EXCESS
MOISTURE

themselves to dust particles that then enter the respiratory system. The hazards of microbial contamination are categorized as either *infectious* or *allergy-inducing*. Infectious diseases are most commonly caused by viruses and bacteria. In 1976, for instance, Legionnaire's disease, caused by the *Legionella pneumophila* bacterium, killed twenty-nine American Legionnaires attending a conference at a Philadelphia hotel, becoming in the process a legendary example of biological pollution. Other diseases spread by airborne infectious agents include respiratory ailments, tuberculosis, smallpox, measles, chicken pox, and staph infections.

Allergic reactions to biological agents are quite widespread. Pollen, molds, mites, dander, and fungi can cause a runny nose, sore throat, watery eyes, sneezing, coughing, and upper respiratory discomfort. Hives or other rashes can develop in sensitive people, and severely allergic individuals and asthmatics can have trouble breathing. With prolonged exposure almost anyone can develop an allergy to a biological agent. Humidifier fever and hypersensitivity pneumonitis, two particularly troublesome, influenzalike responses to microbial contamination characterized by fever, chills, malaise, muscle aches, and sometimes chest tightness, can affect anyone, whether or not the person has a history of other allergies.

The problem of microbial contamination is generally more serious in office buildings and other public spaces than in the home—but not always. After seeing several members of a family with mystifying congestion, fatigue, and confusion, Dr. Robert Jacobs, a scientist with the department of virology at the Southwest Foundation for Biological Research, followed a hunch and went to visit his ailing patients at home. There he found high levels of airborne mold and bacteria that were eventually traced back to a contaminated central air-conditioning system. When the problem was cleared up, the symptoms disappeared.

Testing Procedures

Because high humidity can lead to biological growths that foul indoor air, it is important to monitor the average relative humidity in your home. Inexpensive humidity gauges can be purchased at most local hardware stores. Install them in the bathroom, kitchen, and basement, and get into the habit of checking them regularly.

Unfortunately, there are no easy-to-use, reliable kits available for determining the presence of biological agents. Mold and bacterial spores suspended in indoor air can sometimes be measured with a container specially equipped to support microbial growth. The culture that grows in the monitor can later be identified under a microscope. However, results obtained by this method are of limited value because only the heaviest spores settle into the sample dish, making it impossible to measure spore concentration accurately.

If odors or health effects suggest contamination, use the techniques described below to clear the air. Only if problems linger should you consider having your air tested by a professional laboratory.

Eliminating Biological Agents

Keeping indoor relative humidity levels between 30 and 50 percent in the winter and between 40 and 60 percent in the summer, taking quick action to repair water leaks, eliminating stagnant pools of water before biological agents begin to breed, and maintaining good cleanliness habits are the most effective ways to control microbial growth. Allowing adequate fresh air to circulate through the house, as discussed in the following chapter, is also crucial. In general, it is best to try the easiest, least expensive solutions first; if these don't bring moisture content to an acceptable level, then you can consider more drastic measures.

REDUCE INDOOR HUMIDITY LEVELS: The kitchen, the bath-room, and the basement are the three areas where biological contaminants are most likely to breed, so special attention in these rooms will go a long way toward eliminating microbial agents.

Some specific tips for reducing indoor humidity levels:

- Install exhaust fans vented to the outdoors that are powerful enough to remove moist air quickly from the kitchen and bathroom. Bathroom and kitchen fans can be connected to a humidistat so they switch on when humidity levels build.
- Be sure the clothes dryer is vented to the outdoors. Its warm, moist exhaust increases humidity levels and spews out potentially toxic dust particles that are too small to be intercepted by the machine's lint filter.
- Ventilate your attic and basement crawl space to re-duce excess moisture. Drainage in the basement can be improved with a sump pump or with drain tiles; the latter is expensive to add to a finished house and should be attempted only where there is a severe problem. A polyethylene ground cover can also be placed on top of the soil in the crawl space. In a warm, humid climate, a dehumidifier is an effective way to lower humidity levels.
- Clean the basement floor drain frequently with a dis-infectant to prevent the buildup of microbes.
- Connect your centralized air-to-air heat exchanger to a humidistat so that the system will operate when the moisture level becomes too high.
- If green lumber or wet wood is used for construction projects, extra ventilation should be provided until the wood is thoroughly dry.
- If you are building a new house or an addition, put a vapor retarder under the concrete slab floor and add waterproofing materials to the outside of the founda-tion.

• Use storm windows or double pane windows to control condensation.

REPAIR LEAKS: Leaks in the roof or plumbing system should be repaired promptly. Every drop of water that splashes into the sink or tub from a leaky faucet releases unseen spray into the air. Evaporation from the damp areas around a leaking fixture further contributes to indoor humidity. Even a small leak supports microbial growth and can lead to expensive structural damage.

An overflowing bathtub or sink and other accidental spills can soak carpets, insulation, and building materials with moisture. To prevent mold and bacterial growth from gaining a footing in your house, try to dry such water damage within twenty-four hours. Aiming a portable heater at the wet spots, raising indoor temperatures above normal, and opening some windows to increase ventilation all speed drying. If odors persist or health effects become obvious after the water damage occurs, you may have to replace wet wallboard, insulation, or carpets. It is best to nip microbial growth in the bud because it can be hard to control once it becomes established.

Another way to keep your bathroom moisture-free is to make certain that the ceramic tile or waterproof panels around your bathtub or shower are watertight. The grout between ceramic tiles should be touched up and resealed with liquid silicone every few years. The caulking where the tub or shower makes contact with the bathroom walls and floor also needs to be renewed regularly.

ELIMINATE STANDING WATER: Any source of standing water is a ready breeding ground for microbes. For that reason, condensate trays in the refrigerator, dehumidifier, and air conditioner should all be emptied and disinfected frequently. Clearing out the clogged drain from the central air conditioning unit to the outdoors was all that was necessary to eliminate the contamination that was making Dr. Robert Jacobs's patients so ill.

Cool mist or ultrasonic humidifiers pose particular dangers of microbial contamination and should be avoided unless absolutely necessary for comfort. According to the U.S. Consumer Product Safety Commission, you should take these precautions if you use a humidifier in your home or apartment:

- If possible, change the water on a daily basis so that film and scaly materials do not accumulate. Always dump the old water before adding fresh water.
- Use distilled water, rather than mineral-rich tap water, to reduce the buildup of microorganisms.
- Scrub your humidifiers regularly and replace filters, sponges, or other disposable parts at least as often as recommended by the manufacturer.
- If you must use a cleanser that contains chlorine or another toxic cleaning product, be sure to rinse the tank thoroughly so that you do not inhale harmful chemicals.

USE DEHUMIDIFIERS: Dehumidifiers, which are especially valuable on muggy summer days, are rated according to the amount of water they can remove from room air each day. Capacity typically ranges from about 10 to 50 pints per day; higher capacity units are generally most efficient.

Dehumidifiers contain a fan that moves humid air past two coils. The air is first cooled, which causes moisture to condense and drip into a drain pan or hose at the bottom of the unit. Next, the air passes by a heating coil, where it is rewarmed and blown back into the room. In humid weather a dehumidifier must be emptied at least once a day, so be sure to choose a model with a drip pan that is easy to remove and replace. Scrub the pan regularly with disinfectant to prevent the uncontrolled growth of bacteria and mold. If you use a dehumidifier in a basement with a floor drain, you may be able to remove the drip pan altogether and allow condensate to drain out through a hose.

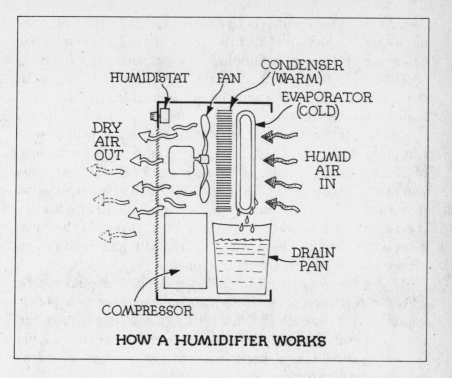

HOW A HUMIDIFIER WORKS

Other important maintenance tips:
- Clean the condenser coils regularly to prevent dust buildup.
- Replace the filter, if your machine has one, at least once a year.
- Oil the fan motor every year, if appropriate. Some motors have sealed bearings that don't require lubrication.

MAINTAIN A CLEAN HOUSE: Good housecleaning habits go a long way to reducing airborne biological contamination. Sheets and pillowcases should be washed regularly in hot water to reduce the presence of mites. Thorough vacuuming and dusting can eliminate household dust, which is typically full of biological contaminants and other toxins.

Unfortunately, running the vacuum can fill the air with dust, so you'll need to open a few windows on housecleaning day. An even better alternative is to purchase a portable vacuum specially designed to filter most of the dust out of exhaust air. If you are building a new house or addition, consider installing a central vacuum system that is vented to the outdoors. Central vacuums are available through most building supply outlets.

AVOID WALL-TO-WALL CARPETING: Replacing wall-to-wall carpeting with hardwood or masonry floors and throw rugs, preferably made of natural fibers, is one of the biggest steps you can take toward better indoor air quality because wood floors and scatter rugs can be cleaned much more effectively. It is particularly important not to cover the floors in the bathroom and kitchen, where water spills and high humidity levels are most likely to attract microbes.

If you do install wall-to-wall carpeting, it should not be placed directly on a concrete slab, unless there is a plastic vapor barrier beneath the concrete. Otherwise, moisture can readily migrate through the slab and into the carpet backing. Carpeting should be cleaned frequently with a pesticide-free solution—ordinary soap and water is best.

TEND TO YOUR HOUSE PLANTS: Healthy plants are less likely to become bug-infested than diseased ones, so fertilize and water your houseplants regularly and provide them with adequate sunlight and fresh air. Spraying the leaves with a mild soap-and-water solution will remove accumulated dust and discourage pests.

4
THE FIRE WITHIN
Combustion Contaminants

Burning anything inside the home consumes life-sustaining oxygen and can contaminate indoor air. One of the worst offenders is cigarettes—some 4,000 different chemicals are present in the tar alone, including a number of confirmed carcinogens. Stoves, space heaters, fireplaces, clothes dryers, and furnaces, whether fueled by charcoal, gas, kerosene, oil, or wood, are all potential sources of indoor pollution. Emissions from a car's idling engine in an attached garage or from traffic on a nearby roadway can also make their way indoors and increase the collection of toxins.

Here's a closer look at three hazardous by-products of the combustion process: carbon monoxide, nitrogen oxides, and respirable suspended particulates.

CARBON MONOXIDE

New Year's Eve, 1989. The temperature had plummeted in Butte, Montana, and all the windows and doors of a local residence were sealed shut. A group of partygoers were enjoying themselves in the house's finished basement. A fire was blazing in the fireplace. It was an innocent enough scene, but before the evening was over, it would turn into a medical emergency.

Because there was insufficient fresh air in the house, the fire became starved for oxygen. The only way for outside air to enter the house was through the exhaust chimney of a natural gas furnace. The fire attempted to pull oxygen through that chimney but succeeded only in drawing carbon monoxide–laden exhaust back into the tightly sealed room. Seven people were overcome by the fumes and rushed to the hospital, where they had to be treated in special oxygen-rich chambers.

The Montana partygoers were relatively lucky—they survived. A family of eight perished in a similar situation in Memphis, Tennessee. While such tragedies are rare, they demonstrate the very real hazards of carbon monoxide poisoning. The problem is called *backdrafting* and it occurs in tightly sealed houses where wood stoves, fireplaces, and furnaces are burning. If sufficient outdoor air cannot infiltrate a home to replace air that is being exhausted, negative pressure builds indoors. Once this negative pressure exceeds the draft of the building's chimney, exhaust gases can be drawn down the chimney and back into the house, poisoning the inhabitants with a sometimes-lethal dose of carbon monoxide.

Carbon monoxide is part of the residue of the combustion process and cannot be seen, sensed, or tasted. While backdrafting is the most catastrophic source of carbon monoxide exposure, it is more commonly emitted from poorly vented gas and kerosene space heaters, wood or coal stoves, poorly maintained gas ranges, cigarette smoke, and automobile emissions. Even at low levels, exposure to carbon monoxide is dangerous and uncomfortable.

What Are the Health Hazards?

Carbon monoxide is absorbed through the lungs into the bloodstream, where it inhibits the ability of the blood to carry oxygen. At low levels, headaches and shortness of breath are common, and people with heart disease may complain of chest pains. Prolonged, low-grade carbon monoxide poisoning can also cause flulike symptoms. Most of these symptoms vanish when an individual leaves a contaminated environment and begins to breathe normal levels of oxygen.

As carbon monoxide concentration mounts, vision and brain function are affected, resulting in confusion, fatigue, nausea, and weakness. Every year a small number of Americans suffocate from intense doses of carbon monoxide.

Carbon Monoxide Concentrations
parts per million (ppm)*

10,000	Human beings exposed to carbon monoxide at this level generally cannot survive longer than ten to twenty minutes.
100	Typical concentration near a busy highway.
50	Unvented kerosene heaters can produce this level of carbon monoxide after forty-five minutes.
35	Environmental Protection Agency standard for maximum allowable outdoor carbon monoxide, averaged over one hour.
15	Indoor exposure at this level for eight hours causes minor confusion and a loss of the sense of time.
10	In Japan, the maximum allowable level for continuous indoor exposure.
9	Environmental Protection Agency standard for maximum allowable outdoor carbon monoxide, averaged over eight hours.
0.5–5	Typical carbon monoxide concentration indoors. Cooking over a gas stove can add another 5 to 10 ppm of carbon monoxide to the air.

*Carbon monoxide is measured in parts per million (ppm). A measurement of 1 ppm indicates that one unit of carbon monoxide is contained in one million units of air.

NITROGEN OXIDES

Nitrogen oxides are among the chief by-products of combustion, produced when gas, oil, or kerosene is burned at high temperatures in the presence of large amounts of oxygen. Nitrogen oxide is relatively benign and is unlikely to pose a health threat, but it rapidly oxidizes to nitrogen dioxide, which is pungent and much more toxic.

The most common household source of nitrogen dioxide is a gas range, used in some 50 percent of American households. The appliance emits nitrogen dioxide from the pilot light and during cooking. In impoverished areas, gas stoves are sometimes used as a source of heat, which also increases nitrogen dioxide levels. A number of studies have shown that the indoor concentration of nitrogen dioxide in homes using gas ranges can be two or three times that of homes using electric ranges. Cigarette smoke is another particularly toxic source of indoor nitrogen dioxide.

What Are the Health Hazards?

Nitrogen dioxide can irritate the skin, eyes, and mucous membranes, with effects that range in severity from a mild burning sensation to severe chest pains, violent coughing, and difficult breathing. Like carbon monoxide, nitrogen dioxide has an attraction to blood hemoglobin, and at high concentrations (much higher than ordinary indoor levels) it can interfere with the blood's capacity to carry oxygen.

The possibility that long-term exposure to nitrogen dioxide ultimately can cause chronic respiratory illness or bronchitis in adults remains a subject of some dispute within the scientific community. A few studies have associated reduced lung function with the use of gas for cooking, but some researchers claim the correlation is imprecise and unproven. Children living in homes with gas ranges have been found to have higher rates of respiratory infection and below-normal pulmonary function, but here, too, scientific findings are somewhat contradictory.

Nitrogen Dioxide Concentrations
parts per million (ppm)*

50	Prolonged exposure at this level is known to cause lung damage and chronic lung disease.
25	Prolonged exposure at this level can cause bronchitis.
5	Occupational Safety and Health Administration standard for workplace exposure, averaged over eight hours.
0.1–0.5	Respiratory irritation likely in individuals with chronic respiratory ailments.
0.12	Level at which gaseous odor can be detected.
0.05	EPA standard for maximum concentration, averaged over one year.
0.025–0.08	Typical concentration found in homes with gas stoves.

*Nitrogen dioxide is measured in parts per million (ppm). A measurement of 1 ppm indicates that one unit of nitrogen dioxide is contained in one million units of air.

RESPIRABLE SUSPENDED PARTICULATES

Respirable suspended particulates (RSPs) are airborne matter small enough to be inhaled deep into the lungs yet large enough to remain lodged once they enter. RSPs come in an enormous variety of sizes, shapes, and levels of toxicity, and much scientific research about their health effects, both singly and in combination with one another, remains undone. Benzo-(a)-pyrene, a tarry, organic chemical that is a product of incomplete combustion, is probably the most studied RSP, and one of the most dangerous.

A few years ago, Environmental Protection Agency employee James L. Repace agreed to carry a monitor equipped to measure RSPs during the course of a day. Although he strolled through downtown Washington, D.C., and sat behind a smoky diesel truck on his commute home, the monitor recorded the highest levels of RSPs as he cooked dinner over his gas stove. The second-highest levels were produced in the smoking section of his office cafeteria.

Repace's story is a dramatic illustration of why indoor combustion is a particular source of concern. Cigarette smoke, wood stoves, fireplaces, kerosene space heaters, gas-fired ranges, furnaces, and water heaters can all introduce significant particles into the air. While not related to combustion, other sources of RSPs include building materials and insulation, home furnishings, microbes, household dust, people, pets, and infiltrating outdoor air.

Automobile and industrial emissions are leading sources of the lead particles inside many homes. While leaded gasoline is gradually being phased out in this country, no-knock additives still contain the metal and vehicle exhaust continues to be a major pollutant. Lead fumes or dust originating from water pipes, paints, inks, and batteries can also enter household air and water through noncombustion processes.

The nose, throat, and bronchial tubes can filter out particles larger than 1.5 microns (a micron is one-millionth of a meter), while particles smaller than 0.1 micron are usually exhaled. Thus the particles of greatest concern are those that range in size from .1 micron to 1.5 microns. No standards have been set for acceptable indoor air concentration levels of RSPs.

What Are the Health Hazards?

The biological, chemical, and physical characteristics of specific particles will determine whether they enter the bloodstream, are washed out of the lungs with mucous, or

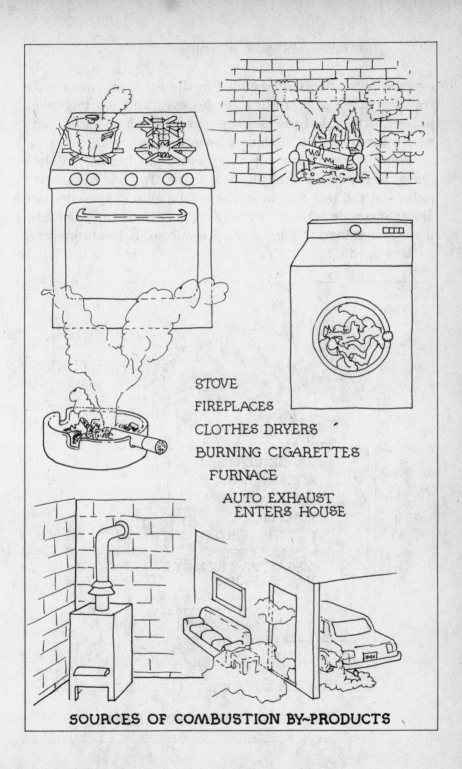

STOVE
FIREPLACES
CLOTHES DRYERS
BURNING CIGARETTES
FURNACE
AUTO EXHAUST
ENTERS HOUSE

SOURCES OF COMBUSTION BY-PRODUCTS

become permanently embedded in the lung. At low concentrations, RSPs are irritants to the eyes and mucous membranes. At higher doses, they are also associated with respiratory illnesses, including bronchitis and emphysema.

Some RSPs are toxic in their own right because of their chemical composition or physical shape. The one trillion particles emitted into the air in the combustion of one cigarette are an example. The risk of lung cancer from cigarette smoking is due at least in part to the presence of benzo-(a)-pyrene, a carcinogenic RSP.

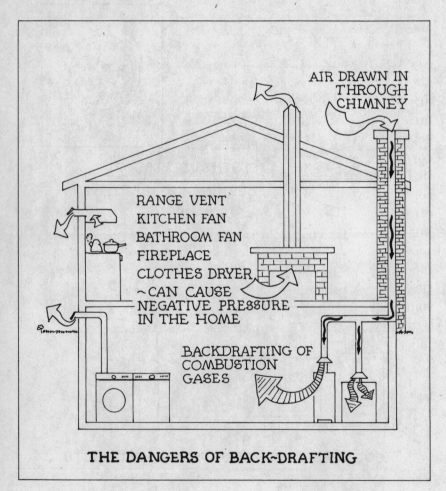

AIR DRAWN IN
THROUGH
CHIMNEY

RANGE VENT
KITCHEN FAN
BATHROOM FAN
FIREPLACE
CLOTHES DRYER
~CAN CAUSE
NEGATIVE PRESSURE
IN THE HOME

BACKDRAFTING OF
COMBUSTION
GASES

THE DANGERS OF BACK-DRAFTING

Asbestos and lead are other especially hazardous particles. Airborne lead targets the brain, kidney, and bone mar-
row when it is ingested or inhaled. Prolonged, low levels of
exposure can result in fatigue, muscle aches and tremors,
headaches, and stomach pain. The consequences of acute,
high-dose lead exposure are more severe, even life-
threatening. Lead poisoning has been associated with retardation, behavioral problems, and cognitive dysfunction in
young children. The toxic metal is also linked to high blood
pressure, acute nervousness, anemia, insomnia, and, in extreme cases, personality changes, kidney and brain damage,
and paralysis.

RSPs that are not hazardous alone become dangerous because they absorb or combine with airborne toxins to create
a particle that is more likely to become lodged deep in the
lungs. For instance, sulfur dioxide, which can impair breathing and is produced when sulfur-containing fuels are burned,
acts synergistically with asbestos, cigarette smoke, soot, and
coal dust, worsening the hazards of each. Carbon dioxide particles emitted from combustion sources are nontoxic by themselves, but they absorb other airborne contaminants
efficiently and can carry these absorbed pollutants into the
lungs.

Pregnant women and young children are, unfortunately,
most at risk. Expectant mothers are at greater risk of miscarriage and a baby carried to term may be born with lead poisoning. Making matters worse, concentrations of lead that
would have no noticeable effect on adults can arrest the
physical and mental development of an infant.

TESTING FOR COMBUSTION BY-PRODUCTS

Relatively inexpensive carbon monoxide and nitrogen dioxide detectors are available. Like formaldehyde monitors,
they typically consist of a glass or plastic tube cannister with

specially treated filter screens at one end. The screens are exposed to indoor air for about one week before the detector is recapped and returned to the lab for analysis. Alarms and other monitoring devices are also available to signal residents when carbon monoxide levels climb too high.

It is much more difficult to analyze respirable suspended particulates because they are so varied and numerous. Highly sophisticated electronic instruments can now measure the nature and concentration of RSPs directly, but equipment costs can easily exceed $500,000. As with volatile organic compounds, there is little reason to go to the considerable expense of having a lab analyze the toxic suspended particles in the air; it is much more practical to follow the control measures outlined here if you suspect a problem.

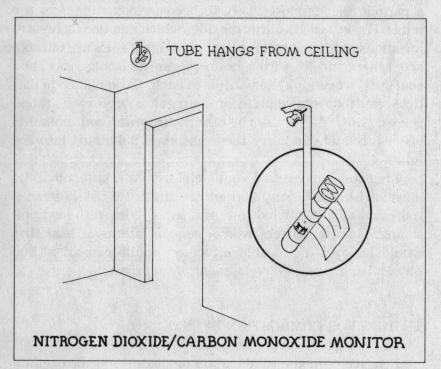

TUBE HANGS FROM CEILING

NITROGEN DIOXIDE/CARBON MONOXIDE MONITOR

ELIMINATING COMBUSTION BY-PRODUCTS

Good ventilation, combined with some of the techniques suggested below, can go a long way to reducing the danger of harmful emissions. One important note: It is almost futile to take these actions if people are still smoking lots of cigarettes inside your home. At the very least, smoking should be confined to one well-ventilated room. Better yet, don't allow any smoking at all indoors.

GAS STOVES: Most of the contaminants from a natural gas or propane stove or oven can be eliminated with proper source ventilation. It is especially crucial to use the vent hood while the stove is on. Here are some other ways to reduce the contamination from gas-cooking equipment:

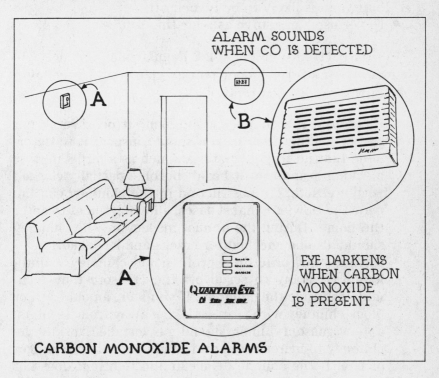

ALARM SOUNDS WHEN CO IS DETECTED

A

B

EYE DARKENS WHEN CARBON MONOXIDE IS PRESENT

QUANTUM EYE

A

CARBON MONOXIDE ALARMS

- Be sure that the flame burns a uniformly blue color. If the flame tip is yellow the combustion process is incomplete and there is likely to be an increased emission of pollutants. The local gas company will usually adjust your stove and oven burners if necessary.
- When you are ready to purchase a new stove or hot water heater, consider the benefits of a clean electric model, especially if you live in a tight, energy-efficient house.
- If you prefer to buy a gas stove, be sure it has electronic igniters rather than pilot lights. About one-third of the gas used by a stove or oven is consumed by pilot lights, which burn all the time, whether or not you are actually cooking. This wastes energy and unnecessarily spews pollutants into the air, especially since the exhaust fan is likely to be turned off.
- Never use a gas stove as a heating source.

WOOD STOVE AND FIREPLACES: Regular maintenance will eliminate most of the indoor contaminants generated by a wood-burning stove or fireplace.

- Be certain the chimney is in good shape. Every year before heating season, you should inspect it to determine that no foreign material (such as a bird's nest) is blocking it and that it hasn't become partially clogged with creosote. An obstruction in the chimney can impede the flow of exhaust gases, allowing fumes to enter the home. During the annual inspection, the chimney should also be checked for cracks and loose mortar.
- Once a year, bring in a professional chimney maintenance company to scrub off the creosote that accumulates inside the chimney. If you have an old brick or block chimney with mortar flaking away from its joints, a new masonry liner should be installed inside the chimney to increase the draft and eliminate the danger of fire. If the chimney is clean and tight but does not exhaust fumes properly, it may have to be extended a few feet higher.

- Inspect your wood-burning stove to see that it is as air-tight as possible. Be certain the loading door fits snugly. If the stove door has a fabric seal, watch for signs of deterioration and replace the seal promptly. The pipe that connects the stove to the chimney or to a metal flue through the wall or ceiling should have no cracks or holes in it. All pipe joints should fit tightly; any flue pipe that shows signs of corrosion should be replaced.
- Burn only well-seasoned wood. Never burn preservative-treated wood, because it will corrode the stove's metal and emit toxic smoke, or colored paper, which releases arsenic vapors.
- Unless outdoor air is piped directly to your stove or fireplace, you should crack open a nearby window to provide adequate combustion air and to avoid back-drafting.
- Don't allow fires to smolder and never completely close the flue before retiring. A hot fire belches far less smoke into outside air, is less likely to pollute an indoor space, and greatly reduces the buildup of creosote inside the chimney. When a fire begins to die down, heat may be insufficient to move exhaust gases out the chimney, especially when outdoor winds are strong. Stir a dying fire thoroughly and keep the flue open to ensure complete combustion of the remaining wood.
- When you are ready to purchase a new wood stove, be certain that it is certified in compliance with federal emission standards. The stove shouldn't be oversized— one that's just big enough to do the job properly will burn more efficiently than a larger model that is not fully loaded with wood.

FURNACES: Furnaces fueled by natural gas, propane, or heating oil should be inspected before they are put into service at the start of each heating season. The chimney and the pipes running from the furnace to the chimney should be examined for obstructions, holes, cracks, or corrosion. Begin the heating season with a fresh filter and replace it about once a month while the furnace is in use. Any other service and maintenance instructions from the furnace manufacturer should be followed carefully.

SPACE HEATERS: Because so many fatal fires and incidents of carbon monoxide poisoning have been attributed to portable gas and kerosene space heaters, many local fire and safety codes now ban their use. The models that remain on the market, however, have been substantially improved over those available a decade ago—they emit far less pollution and the fire hazard has been reduced. The key to the safe use of space heaters is proper ventilation—you should keep the room door to the rest of the house ajar and open a window slightly. Be certain your space heater burns with an entirely blue flame and follow all manufacturer's instructions.

AUTOMOBILES: Much of the lead contamination in household air originates with automobile emissions. Fortunately, the alarming discoveries during the 1980s about the effects of even minute quantities of lead on nervous system development has heightened the pressure to remove it from the human environment. The widespread use of unleaded gasoline is an important step in this direction.

If you have an attached garage, several important precautions can minimize the risk of carbon monoxide poisoning:

- Leave the garage door open for a few minutes after parking your car to allow exhaust and engine fumes to disperse.
- Never allow the car to idle inside the garage with the doors closed. If you warm up the car in the morning, be sure to pull it out of the garage first.
- Make sure the wall and doorway separating the garage from your house are airtight. Weather stripping and the threshold around the entry door should be in good shape, and a continuous vapor barrier should be installed on the indoor side of the wall separating the garage from the house.

5
A PROPER AIRING
The Science
of Ventilation

Historically, atmospheric pollutants have been regulated by the maxim "Dilution is the solution to pollution." In other words, if contaminants are mixed with enough fresh air, the threat to the outdoor environment will be minimized. In this age of photochemical smog, acid rain, and global air pollution, this theory no longer has much validity outside, but it is still a good guideline for improving the quality of indoor air. In addition to employing the techniques of source control described in earlier chapters, providing adequate ventilation in your home will go a long way toward reducing high indoor humidity and the concentration of airborne toxic substances.

But what can you do to assure adequate airflow? Throw open the windows year-round, pay exorbitant heating and cooling bills, and breathe easier knowing that at least you are investing in clear air? Fortunately, no. Today, there are better ways to enjoy the draft-free comfort and low heating bills associated with a tightly built home while maintaining good air quality. Here's a look at how to boost the circulation of fresh air through your home with natural and mechanical ventilation.

NATURAL VENTILATION

Natural ventilation is the unaided movement of air into and out of the house. It includes *infiltration*, outside air passing through cracks into the home; *exfiltration*, the corresponding movement of air out of the house; and the passage of air through open windows and doors. Natural ventilation rates are determined by temperature differences between indoor and outdoor air, by differences in temperature within the house, and by wind. As a result, natural ventilation rates will vary widely, depending on weather, the location and orientation of your home, and the position of windows and doors.

How Can I Boost Natural Ventilation?

You can enhance air circulation through your house or apartment by adopting many of the following suggestions:

- Leave interior doors open when possible. By improving internal circulation, you can prevent airborne contaminants from building up in closed rooms and stop wet spots that harbor microorganisms from developing.
- Open your windows. Even in the coldest and hottest parts of the country, there are several months a year when fresh outdoor air can comfortably circulate through the house.
- Make sure your windows are in good working order. If they tend to stick or won't stay open, it may seem like too much trouble to use them.
- Add screen doors, if your home doesn't already have them. Combination screen and storm doors are the best because the storm window can be closed during the hottest and coldest seasons to keep your utility bills low but kept open during mild weather to allow fresh air to circulate.
- Clean window and door screens regularly to increase airflow. Be sure to inspect the screens periodically for small tears that might allow insects inside.

Even better, do any remodeling or new construction with ventilation in mind. While you may have to spend a little more time in the planning stages, additional building costs should be negligible. Generally, homeowners can implement the suggestions that follow more readily than renters. However, if you are a tenant, you may be able to interest the landlord in making some needed changes, especially if you emphasize the prospect of increasing property values.

- Remove interior walls. Many older homes are divided into separate living room, dining room, and kitchen areas that obstruct air circulation. By removing walls to open up interior spaces, you can enhance air circulation and often improve the aesthetics of your environment at the same time.

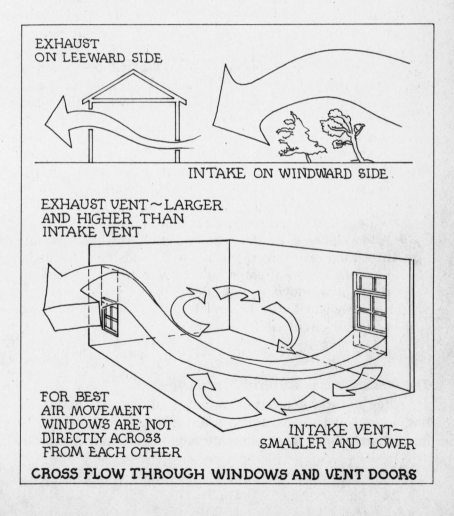

EXHAUST ON LEEWARD SIDE

INTAKE ON WINDWARD SIDE

EXHAUST VENT ~ LARGER AND HIGHER THAN INTAKE VENT

FOR BEST AIR MOVEMENT WINDOWS ARE NOT DIRECTLY ACROSS FROM EACH OTHER

INTAKE VENT ~ SMALLER AND LOWER

CROSS FLOW THROUGH WINDOWS AND VENT DOORS

- Provide adequate clearance under the doors. Internal circulation is improved by removing at least one inch of the wood framework on the bottom of every door. Although most inside doors have hollow cores, removing an inch of framework won't weaken the door.
- Cut openings above interior doors. A hole as wide as the door, from eight to twelve inches high, and located as close to the ceiling as possible, will allow the rising warm air to flow out of the room. You may want to cover the opening with louvers or a decorative screen. Older houses often have transom windows above the doors that can be restored by scraping away accumulated paint and replacing hinges and latches as needed.
- Add windows or special vent doors. The best circulation occurs if windows are located on opposite walls, but not directly across from one another. If the wind in your area most frequently comes out of the west, opening windows on the east and west walls of the house will ensure even cross-ventilation. Insulated vent doors can also be installed near the floor on windward walls and near the ceiling on leeward walls. Vent doors cost less, lose less heat, and are more effective than windows in enhancing air circulation.
- Add a ceiling vent. An exhaust vent at the highest point in a room can pull rising warm air outside. The slight vacuum that is created helps draw fresh air back in through windows or vent doors in the walls. An operable skylight located above the room's ceiling can also boost air circulation.

The Limitations of Natural Ventilation

While natural ventilation improves indoor air quality, it has several limitations. Infiltration, in particular, is a fairly inefficient way to keep contaminants out of your home because air is not uniformly distributed and the flow cannot be readily controlled.

The air that moves constantly through the building shell does not circulate evenly, so stale air invariably collects in some dead spaces while an abundance of ventilation elsewhere sends heating and cooling costs soaring. Also, infiltration is dirty because exterior walls trap particles of pollen and dust as outdoor air passes through. In a drafty home, this dust accumulates and on a windy day it is likely to be blown indoors.

Because of these drawbacks, it is economical to limit infiltration with energy conservation measures—such as weather-stripping, putting loose windowpanes, and adding storm doors—and to use a combination of controlled natural ventilation, as outlined above, and mechanical ventilation to supply fresh air to your home.

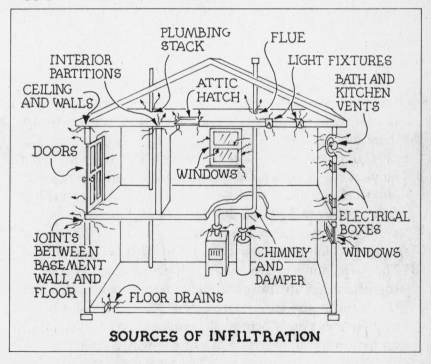

SOURCES OF INFILTRATION

MECHANICAL VENTILATION

Mechanical ventilation systems use electric fans and blowers to pull fresh air inside, to circulate air through a house or apartment, and to exhaust stale indoor air. Bathroom and kitchen exhaust fans, air-to-air heat exchangers, and heat pump ventilators are all types of mechanical ventilation used to maintain good indoor air quality. Ceiling fans, which have become popular in recent years, simply recirculate indoor air; this helps to reduce dampness caused by condensation but has little effect on the concentration of contaminants.

The need for good ventilation results partly from the widespread use of central heating and air-conditioning systems. While both are marvelously convenient—indeed, little

Technical Talk

The ventilation business uses two terms to measure the rate of air movement: air changes per hour (ac/h) and cubic feet per minute (cf/m). Recommended ventilation rates are generally given in ac/h, while mechanical ventilation equipment is rated in cf/m, so you need to understand both terms.

Cubic feet per minute is a measure of the rate of air movement. A bathroom exhaust fan is usually rated at less than 100 cf/m. Whole-house ventilation systems will move between 150 and 500 cf/m of air.

The *air changes per hour* figure represents the average rate at which indoor air is replaced by fresh outdoor air. The ac/h numbers are rough guidelines based on the assumption that air flows through a home evenly, although that's rarely the case. More often, some parts of a house or apartment are fairly well ventilated, while very little air moves through certain out-of-the-way corners.

short of miraculous from the viewpoint of generations past— they can be associated with a variety of air quality problems. In a centralized system, a network of ducts is used to deliver heated and cooled air to each room. Because the system is designed to serve the whole house, opening a window for fresh air in one room can adversely affect the system's over- all performance. In addition, temperature and air circulation rates can rarely be controlled in individual rooms, despite the fact that needs vary widely. Worse, in most modern apartment buildings, individual tenants have little or no control over the heating and cooling systems in their own apartments.

Another problem with centralized temperature control systems is that they allow only a small percentage of fresh air into the building at any one time. Most systems typically

---

In a typically well-insulated new home, infiltration al- lows about one air change per hour. In an ultratight, superinsulated home, the ac/h figure plunges to about one-tenth this rate, while in a drafty house, infiltration and exfiltration can push rates as high as 2 to 10 ac/h. Optimal air change rates depend on the pollu- tion sources that are present in a house or apartment.

If you know the volume of an indoor space and the optimal number of air changes per hour, you can calcu- late the number of cubic feet per minute of fresh air needed to provide adequate ventilation. Let's say you own a 2,000-square-foot home with 8-foot ceilings, mak- ing the total volume of space in your home 16,000 cubic feet. Thirty-two thousand cubic feet of fresh air will thus be needed to obtain 2 air changes per hour. The formula to determine cf/m is simple: 32,000 cubic feet/60 min- utes = 533 cf/m.

recirculate from 80 to 100 percent of indoor air, relying largely on infiltration for the introduction of additional fresh air. Yet research shows that indoor pollution would be minimized if all the stale air in the house or apartment were dumped periodically and replaced with fresh air. Few heating and cooling systems available in the United States are capable of doing this.

Given these limitations, a system of mechanical ventilation is often crucial to air quality, especially in tightly sealed, energy-efficient buildings.

Residential Ventilation Rates

These are the minimum ventilation rates acceptable for residential areas under ASHRAE Standard 62-1989, a voluntary guideline established by the American Society of Heating, Refrigeration and Air-conditioning Engineers.

Residential Area	Cubic Feet per Minute (cf/m)
Living area	15 per person
Kitchen	100 intermittent, or 25 continuous
Bathroom	50 intermittent, or 20 continuous
Garage	100 per car

Source Ventilation

Ventilating at the source of a contaminant can dramatically reduce the need to introduce a fresh supply of outdoor air or to circulate air through the rest of the home. Most, although not all, of the moisture and pollutants carried in indoor air originate from the kitchen and bathroom, so a stove vent hood in the kitchen and an exhaust blower in the bathroom can improve air quality immensely. Without source ventilation, for example, ridding a house of pollutants generated from a gas range requires seven complete air changes per hour (ac/h) in the kitchen. Installing a stove hood, however, pulls pollutants from the house before they mix with the rest of the kitchen air, reducing the rate to a more typical 0.5 to 1 ac/h.

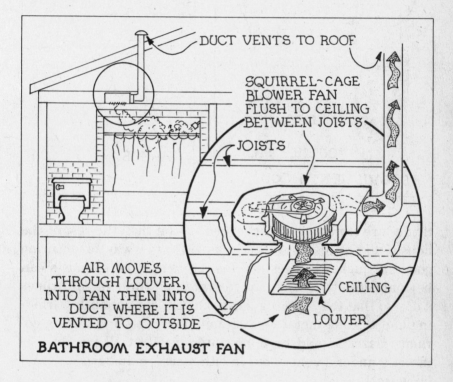

DUCT VENTS TO ROOF

SQUIRREL-CAGE BLOWER FAN FLUSH TO CEILING BETWEEN JOISTS

JOISTS

AIR MOVES THROUGH LOUVER, INTO FAN THEN INTO DUCT WHERE IT IS VENTED TO OUTSIDE

CEILING

LOUVER

BATHROOM EXHAUST FAN

A good way to provide periodic ventilation is to use a timer or to install a humidistat that automatically turns on the kitchen or bathroom exhaust when the humidity reaches a preset level. The exhaust fan should also be run while the kitchen or bathroom is being used and for another ten to fifteen minutes afterwards.

Workshops, hobby centers, and areas where paints or pes-

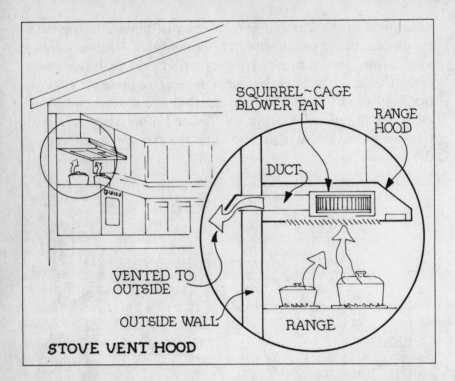

SQUIRREL~CAGE
BLOWER FAN

RANGE
HOOD

DUCT

VENTED TO
OUTSIDE

OUTSIDE WALL

RANGE

STOVE VENT HOOD

ticides are stored need better ventilation than the rest of the house, and an exhaust fan is an effective way of ensuring good air quality in these rooms. Storage room exhausts can be connected to a timer set to switch on three or four times a day so that they run regularly, but not continuously. Grinding and buffing metal and ceramic materials and mixing ceramic glazes should be done outdoors, if at all possible, or directly under a vent hood. In either case, a dust mask should be worn.

Buy the quietest exhaust system available so you won't be reluctant to use it. Squirrel cage blowers, which move air with many small blades located on the outside of a spinning wheel, are generally better than the traditional fans that use three or four large blades. Look for a label from the Underwriters' Laboratories (UL) or the Home Ventilating Institute (HVI), which means the manufacturer voluntarily has had the equipment certified for safety and performance. Ventilation equipment should be installed on flexible mounts to reduce vibration noise. Mounting the fan at the outdoor end of ducting, as far from the living space as possible, also reduces irritating indoor noise.

If you live in an area with cold winters, source ventilation can create problems. When warm, moist air is blown out of the house through cold ducting, water condenses inside the ducts. Frost can even accumulate as the temperatures drop. Ducts that run up from the ceiling to the outdoors can allow

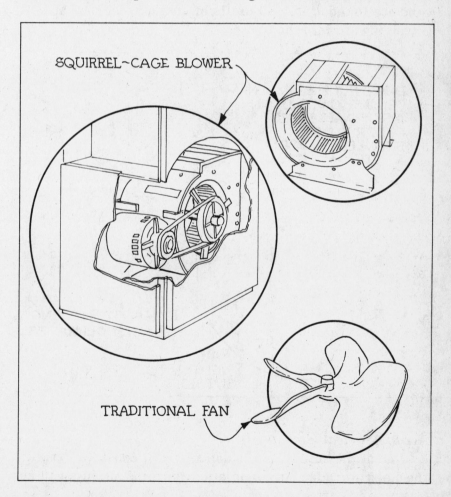

SQUIRREL-CAGE BLOWER

TRADITIONAL FAN

this accumulated water to drip back into the house, while ducts routed through a wall allow it to run down the outside, causing a dark stain. In addition, cold outdoor air can enter the house through the ducting when the exhaust blower isn't running.

To avoid the problem of condensation and cold drafts, exhaust ducts should run down through the floor and outside above the top of the house's foundation. That way, most of the ducting won't be exposed to cold air, condensation will be minimized, excess moisture will drip outdoors onto the concrete foundation, and drafts of cold air won't be able to travel upward into the house.

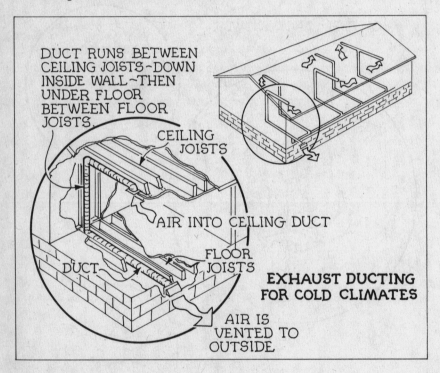

DUCT RUNS BETWEEN CEILING JOISTS~DOWN INSIDE WALL~THEN UNDER FLOOR BETWEEN FLOOR JOISTS.

CEILING JOISTS

AIR INTO CEILING DUCT

FLOOR JOISTS

DUCT

EXHAUST DUCTING FOR COLD CLIMATES

AIR IS VENTED TO OUTSIDE

Air-to-Air Heat Exchangers

One of the best ways to balance energy conservation with the need for adequate ventilation is to install an air-to-air heat exchanger. This mechanical ventilation device blows stale, warm indoor air out of the house, in the process transferring heat to fresh air as it is pulled inside. Heat exchangers do not actually produce heat; they simply move it from one stream of air to another. They can also precool incoming air during the summer, although they are seldom used for this task.

Air-to-air heat exchangers have been widely used in Europe and Canada for more than a decade but have been introduced in American homes only relatively recently. Because high infiltration rates impair the equipment's efficiency, air-to-air heat exchangers are most commonly installed in tightly insulated homes.

HOW THEY WORK: Air-to-air heat exchangers can be either small wall-mounted units or whole-house systems with ducts and vents similar to those used in a central heating and cooling system. The smaller units, which are designed to provide fresh air to one or two rooms or to a small apartment, are about the size of a room air conditioner, cost about $300, and generally deliver less than 100 cubic feet per minute (cf/m) of air. A wall-mounted heat exchanger supplements, but does not substitute for, source ventilation—the bathroom and kitchen still need to be well vented with exhaust fans.

A central system can be the size of a small furnace and will deliver up to 500 cf/m. If you plan for an air-to-air heat exchanger while building a new house or addition, the cost, including installation, should run about $2,000. The cost of installing a central system in an existing home is usually considerably higher. A central air-to-air heat exchanger system is hooked up to every room in the house, via a system of ducts, so no additional source ventilation is necessary.

Within the housing of either type of air-to-air heat exchanger are a heat exchanger core, two fans, controls, a defrosting mechanism, and a condensate drain. When the fans are turned on, air is propelled through the cardboard, plastic, or metal core, which transfers about 70 percent of the heat contained in the stale outgoing air to the fresh airstream. As the stale air is cooled, its capacity to hold water decreases, and condensation accumulates and runs out the drain. The defroster is used to melt the ice that can build inside the equipment during the winter, hindering heat transfer and eventually blocking the passage of air.

When shopping for an air-to-air heat exchanger, be sure to hear it running before making a final selection because some of the equipment can be quite noisy. You should also

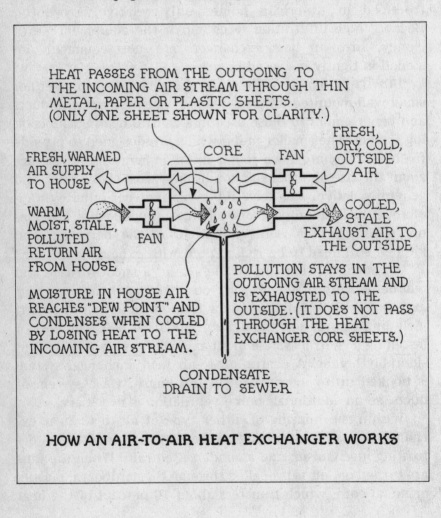

HEAT PASSES FROM THE OUTGOING TO
THE INCOMING AIR STREAM THROUGH THIN
METAL, PAPER OR PLASTIC SHEETS.
(ONLY ONE SHEET SHOWN FOR CLARITY.)

FRESH, WARMED
AIR SUPPLY
TO HOUSE

CORE   FAN

FRESH,
DRY, COLD,
OUTSIDE
AIR

WARM,
MOIST, STALE,
POLLUTED
RETURN AIR
FROM HOUSE

FAN

COOLED,
STALE
EXHAUST AIR TO
THE OUTSIDE

MOISTURE IN HOUSE AIR
REACHES "DEW POINT" AND
CONDENSES WHEN COOLED
BY LOSING HEAT TO THE
INCOMING AIR STREAM.

POLLUTION STAYS IN THE
OUTGOING AIR STREAM AND
IS EXHAUSTED TO THE
OUTSIDE. (IT DOES NOT PASS
THROUGH THE HEAT
EXCHANGER CORE SHEETS.)

CONDENSATE
DRAIN TO SEWER

HOW AN AIR-TO-AIR HEAT EXCHANGER WORKS

keep in mind the three factors that have a major effect on performance:

- The amount of heat-exchange surface in the core. The greater the surface area, the more heat that can be transferred.
- The speed of airflow within the core. More heat is transferred when the air passes through slowly.
- The direction of the airflow. *Counter-flow* heat exchangers, in which ingoing and outgoing airstreams

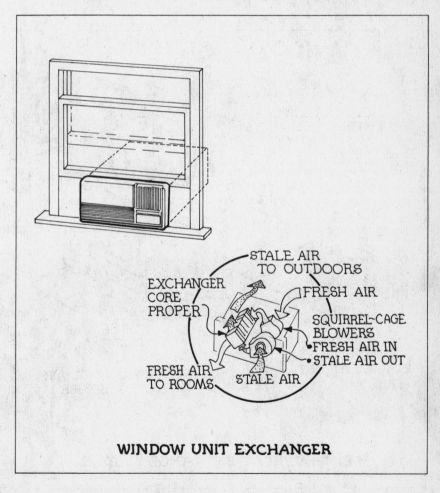

WINDOW UNIT EXCHANGER

move in opposite directions, are generally more efficient than *cross-flow* units, in which the air currents pass each other perpendicularly. Least efficient is a *parallel-flow* core, in which the airstreams move in the same direction.

Note: Don't expect your air-to-air heat exchanger to work quite as efficiently as the manufacturer's specifications suggest. Resistance cuts the fan's capacity: A fan that can move 400 cf/m in open air might move no more than 200 cf/m when

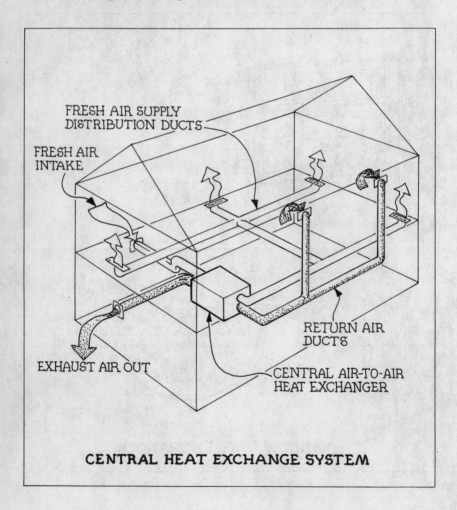

FRESH AIR SUPPLY
DISTRIBUTION DUCTS

FRESH AIR
INTAKE

RETURN AIR
DUCTS

EXHAUST AIR OUT

CENTRAL AIR-TO-AIR
HEAT EXCHANGER

CENTRAL HEAT EXCHANGE SYSTEM

installed. Reputable manufacturers will provide figures for both open air and installed performance.

INSTALLATION AND MAINTENANCE: Properly installing an air-to-air heat exchanger is crucial to efficient performance. If the intake and exhaust vents are positioned too closely together, fresh air entering the house can pass directly back out the exhaust side. Improper installation can also exacerbate a noise problem. You may be able to install a wall-mounted unit yourself, but a central system usually requires the services of a professional.

A heat exchanger also needs to be carefully maintained. Dust from both indoor and outdoor air can accumulate in the system's core and has to be removed regularly. Many systems use air filters, which slightly reduce equipment efficiency, to keep dust out of the core and to remove many of the small toxic particles from incoming air. Other systems use a core that can be removed for cleaning. Replacing filters or cleaning the core at least as often as the manufacturer recommends ensures an efficient operation and prolongs the life of the system.

Heat Pump Ventilators

Heat pumps have become popular over the last twenty years because they provide heat in the winter and cool the air in the summer yet use much less power than resistance electrical heating systems. Used in most government-financed housing in Sweden for years, a heat pump ventilator is a substitute for an air-to-air heat exchanger, a hot water heater, and a dehumidifier. Increasingly it is being used in American homes to heat domestic hot water while maintaining good air quality.

The ventilator pump operates much like a refrigerator or an air conditioner: A liquid with a very low boiling point is circulated through an evaporator coil, where it is vaporized by heat in air that is blown around the coil. The vaporized

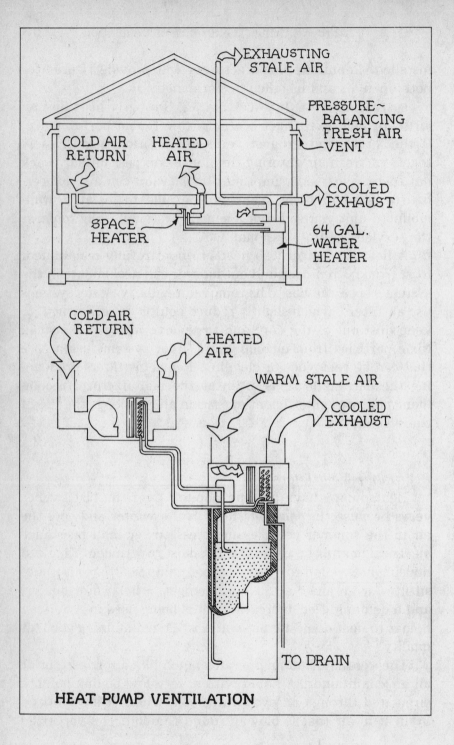

EXHAUSTING
STALE AIR

PRESSURE~
BALANCING
FRESH AIR
VENT

COLD AIR
RETURN

HEATED
AIR

COOLED
EXHAUST

SPACE
HEATER

64 GAL.
WATER
HEATER

COLD AIR
RETURN

HEATED
AIR

WARM STALE AIR

COOLED
EXHAUST

TO DRAIN

HEAT PUMP VENTILATION

refrigerant is piped to a pump, where it is compressed, boosting its temperature. The hot gas then flows through pipes to another heat exchanger, where it is cooled until it recondenses, releasing absorbed energy. The cycle is completed as the liquefied refrigerant passes back to the evaporator coil.

In winter, the heat pump ventilator extracts the heat from stale indoor air before it is exhausted outside. This heat is first used to provide hot water; once the water heater is up to maximum temperature, it is directed instead toward warming the house. In warmer weather, the blower pulls in fresh outdoor air, cools it through the system's evaporating coils, and circulates it through the house. The heat that is removed is again transferred to the hot water heater.

AIR PURIFIERS

The literature for air-cleaning devices makes some bold claims: "Just plug it in, and your problems with indoor dust, pollens, odors, and airborne toxins will be over," and "Filters out virtually everything in the air except the air itself."

Unfortunately, these claims are just not true. The greatest weakness of air purifiers is that they remove only airborne particles—once dust, pollen, or other contaminants settle to the ground, the devices are ineffective. Scientists have concluded that air purifiers do not help individuals suffering from allergies or respiratory disease and are also largely ineffective against toxic gases. Worse, the radon threat can actually be intensified when air cleaners are used. Ordinarily, radon attaches itself to dust particles in the air and becomes heavy enough to settle but when the dust is removed, the radon remains airborne, and therefore inhalable, for a longer period of time.

Does that mean air-cleaning equipment is totally useless? Not quite. According to a February 1989 product review in *Consumer Reports*, the best air purifiers can reduce the irritation from tobacco smoke and remove airborne dust and pollen in one or two rooms. While the review concludes that ventilation is generally the most effective way to purify indoor air, it also says: "If you can't open a window—because the outside air is polluted or the weather is bitter cold—or if you need to ventilate a windowless space, an air purifier may be the only way to reduce smoke and airborne dust."

Air-cleaning devices are available as either tabletop models or room models. Generally, the larger devices are more effective, even when they run at a lower setting. However, they are also more cumbersome, typically weighing about 40 pounds. Smaller models can remove particles only from a small room and then only when operating at top speed. Don't forget to consider the noise factor when making purchasing decisions. No matter how effective the device is, you won't use it regularly if it sounds like a truck on the freeway. Be sure to ask for a demonstration and listen carefully for irritating whines, whirs, or buzzes while the machine runs at various speeds. You can expect to pay anywhere from under $100 to more than $600 for the equipment and will probably have to go to a surgical and medical supply store, a local heating or plumbing contactor, or a regional distributor for the purchase since many retail outlets don't carry them. Some doctors prescribe air purifiers to patients and many also sell them from their offices. Often, these products will be covered by insurance.

Three different methods are used to purify the air: mechanical filtration, electrostatic precipitation, and negative ion generation. *Consumer Reports'* brand name evaluation of air-cleaning devices concluded that high-efficiency particle-arresting (HEPA) filters, used in mechanical filtration, and electrostatic air cleaners are generally the most effective at clearing both smoke and dust from the air.

MECHANICAL FILTERS: The most effective mechanical filter is the HEPA model, composed of tightly packed fibers. Developed during World War II to filter radioactive dust from

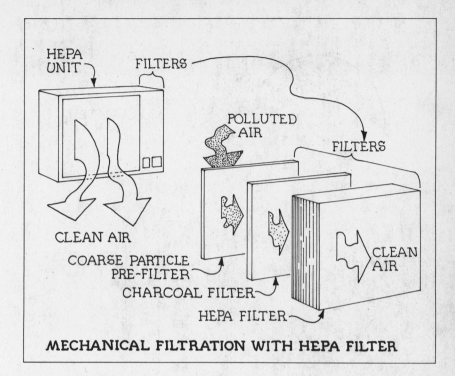

MECHANICAL FILTRATION WITH HEPA FILTER

the exhaust of nuclear fuel plants, HEPA filters can remove all but the tiniest airborne particles. Air may pass first through a prefilter and a porous filter of activated carbon to eliminate certain gaseous particles. An HEPA filter element must be replaced every year or two, at a cost of $50 to $100.

Other mechanical filters use a more loosely packed synthetic fiber medium that removes only larger suspended particles. Such filters generally cost less than HEPA units, but filter elements must be replaced more frequently.

ELECTROSTATIC AIR CLEANERS: These air cleaners transfer an electrical charge to particles in the air. The air then passes over a metal plate with an opposite electrical charge, which works like a magnet to pull out the pollutants. The plates normally need to be removed and washed monthly, so you should choose an electrostatic air purifier with plates that are readily accessible.

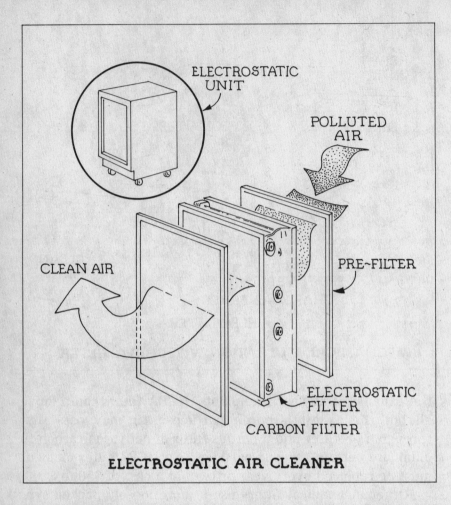

ELECTROSTATIC
UNIT

POLLUTED
AIR

CLEAN AIR

PRE~FILTER

ELECTROSTATIC
FILTER

CARBON FILTER

ELECTROSTATIC AIR CLEANER

NEGATIVE ION GENERATORS: A negative ion generator operates by sending a high voltage across fine needles or wires, ionizing air molecules. These charged molecules then attract airborne particulates, which are usually filtered out or precipitated on a charged surface. Most ionizers have filters, which need to be changed periodically, or collecting plates, which have to be washed. Relatively few manufacturers make ionizers, and the generators are not considered very effective.

HOUSE PLANTS: A simple yet effective natural filtration

method involves keeping plants in your home. In their search for ways to purify the air in space stations, scientists at the National Aeronautics and Space Administration (NASA) discovered that certain houseplants can filter formaldehyde, benzene, carbon monoxide, and nitrous oxides. The process is simple: As schoolchildren know, plants pull carbon dioxide from the air and return oxygen and water vapor as part of the photosynthetic process. More recently, scientists have discovered that other gases are extracted from the air at the same time.

Curiously, some plants are more effective than others at purging the air of particular contaminants. For example, spider plants have an affinity for carbon monoxide; the elephant ear and heart leaf philodendron can absorb large quantities of formaldehyde, benzene, and carbon monoxide; aloe vera is especially good at lowering formaldehyde levels, even at low concentrations; and chrysanthemums and certain species of the common daisy are most useful for removing benzene from the air.

Scattering plants throughout your home is likely to make only a small contribution to clear air because the filtering mechanism is most effective in a tightly sealed environment, but it is an easy and pleasant technique. A more ambitious approach is to redirect your air circulation system through an attached greenhouse, an enclosed window greenhouse, or a solarium, if you are lucky enough to have one.

THE HOUSE OF THE FUTURE

Can we expect the house of the future to be tightly sealed yet provide ample ventilation to control indoor humidity and the buildup of airborne contaminants? Ever since the energy crisis of the 1970s, many builders have assumed so, but one innovative Montana contractor thinks it's not good enough. Steve Loken, owner of South Wall Builders, in Missoula, Montana, has been constructing superinsulated houses since they first came into vogue in the early 1980s. Most have conformed to the accepted formula: heavy insulation, an ultra-tight vapor barrier, and an air-to-air heat exchanger for ventilation.

But Loken never liked the idea of forcing his clients to live in a tightly sealed box that required mechanical ventilation. He also was concerned that if the vapor barrier failed as it grew older, as some experts predict, energy efficiency would plummet. Instead, Loken became an American pioneer of a technique called Fiberglass Canada, developed by the Canadian National Research Council.

This building system features "breathable walls" and a heat pump ventilator that warms domestic hot water with the energy in the stale air being removed from the house. The heat pump maintains a slight vacuum inside the house. Combined with a number of other construction materials, including high-density fiberglass board, fiberglass insulation, and lap siding, the vacuum allows air to enter through the walls slowly and evenly, rather than in cold drafts through cracks, the process normally associated with infiltration. A vapor barrier is installed only between the house and the garage, where it prevents the migration of carbon monoxide and other poisonous gases from automobile exhaust.

Maintaining negative pressure in a house can be dangerous, as we pointed out earlier in this book, because it allows flue gases to be sucked back down the chimney and radon to be pulled into the house from surrounding soil. In Loken's design, however, there are no furnaces, fireplaces, or wood stoves and no basement through which radon can enter. Instead, the house is heated with "radiant floors"—electric heating cables that run through lightweight concrete floors. The cables heat the floors during winter, allowing an even warmth to radiate throughout the house. South-facing windows further temper the house in cold weather. When there is no demand for hot water, the heat pump also blows warm fresh air inside.

Experimenting with such innovative building designs, which make miserly use of energy while providing adequate ventilation and good indoor air quality, is imperative. Neither the problems of indoor pollution nor concerns about outdoor air quality, acid rain, and the global warming trends associated with the greenhouse effect are likely to disappear quickly. Unless new and creative construction solutions are found, the consumer ultimately will pay a high price, in both energy and health costs.

6
NOT A DROP TO DRINK
Keeping Your Water Safe

Bad news about drinking water has become routine. Dire headlines warn that the nation's groundwater is being polluted by agricultural chemicals, industrial solvents, and petroleum products. At the same time, lakes and streams are being tainted by a host of chemicals with difficult-to-pronounce names and alarming health effects. The result is that the clear water that flows from the kitchen tap is likely to carry dangerous—and often hard-to-detect—substances.

Many of the toxic materials used in our industrial society have a perverse way of gaining entry to the water supply. Despite elaborate chemical treatment—and sometimes because of it—we cannot afford to take the purity of drinking water for granted. But there are steps we can take to protect ourselves. By learning how unsafe substances get into the water and what the associated dangers are, and by performing appropriate tests and installing efficient purification systems, we can gain substantial control over one of nature's most irreplaceable resources.

THERE'S NO ESCAPING THE HAZARDS

The World Health Organization (WHO) estimates that more than ten million people die each year from waterborne diseases. Seventy-five percent of the disease in developing countries is the result of unsanitary water systems, according to WHO. While devastating epidemics are no longer carried through the water system in this country, water pollution in

114

the United States poses more subtle hazards and remains an important priority for health and environmental activists.

Bad drinking water is not a problem confined to urban areas, although the sheer volume of people, cars, businesses, and industry might suggest that all forms of pollution are worse in the cities. Ironically, there is actually more water pollution, per capita, in rural regions of this country. One reason is that the mammoth amounts of sewage and garbage generated in densely populated regions simply force efficient disposal. In addition, more money is generally available in cities to dispose of waste properly, to monitor water quality, to enforce pollution laws, and to clean up contaminated water.

By contrast, the fiscal condition in most rural areas is often precarious. In addition, people are more likely to make their living extracting and processing natural resources, such as crops, livestock, minerals, and timber, which often exact a heavy toll on water quality. Erosion from farms and forests clogs streams with silt, salts, herbicides, and insecticides, while mining fouls nearby waters with toxic heavy metals, radioactive wastes, and process chemicals. Leaking underground storage tanks, septic tanks, and wells and illegally dumped toxic materials further degrade rural water quality. Even the most remote and apparently pristine bodies of water in sparsely populated areas can be poisoned by airborne pesticides, acid rain, and disease-carrying organisms.

SURFACE WATER AND ITS CONTAMINANTS

The American landscape is graced with two million miles of streams and almost 80,000 square miles of lakes and reservoirs. This surface water quenches about half the nation's thirst for drinking water, with the remainder coming from groundwater sources (discussed in the next section).

But numerous industrial processes and accidents threaten the purity of surface water. Manufacturing plants, mines, and smelters can all taint. Train derailments and automobile and marine disasters often result in dangerous runoffs that make their way into the drinking water system. Raw sewage and toxic industrial chemicals spill far too frequently into lakes and rivers. And the sediments in riverbeds and on the banks of lakes and streams are commonly found to be loaded with toxic wastes that have accumulated over a period of many years.

Along with centralized sources of pollution, such as factories and toxic waste dumps, there are literally tens of thousands of diffuse pollutants. Some examples: runoff from streets and parking lots, which can contain lead, salts, oil, and gasoline; eroding soil and pesticides from forests and farmlands; even the backyard use and disposal of lawn and garden chemicals.

A further problem is that, in recent years, the high demand for water, combined with severe droughts, have depleted the level of many lakes and streams. Poor water quality is one enduring result, partly because less water is available to dilute any contaminants. In addition, high water temperatures result from falling water levels, which can upset the biological balance of a body of water, and kill fish. This damage takes years to repair.

Signs of Progress

The deplorable condition of the nation's lakes and rivers was one catalyst for the environmental activism that arose during the 1960s. After more than a century's service as a repository for wastes, too many rivers had been reduced to little more than open sewers. Fish could no longer survive in the most polluted waters, and no-swimming signs dotted public beaches from coast to coast. A public outcry eventually forced Congress to take note, and two groundbreaking pieces of legislation—the Clean Water Act of 1972 and the Safe Drinking Water Act of 1974—were enacted into law. (See Appendix, "Key Federal Air and Water Legislation," page 221.)

A total of $125 billion has since been appropriated to construct municipal sewer facilities, with another $75 billion targeted for industrial waste treatment plants. According to a 1989 report by the Office of Technology Assessment, an additional $500 billion in government and private funds will be spent over the next fifty years to clean up Superfund sites, the waste sites designated by the EPA as the nation's most toxic.

Although the EPA estimates it will cost an additional $83.5 billion just to upgrade sewage treatment plants to comply with the Clean Water Act, the monies spent to date have made an enormous difference. Better waste treatment facilities and the efforts to contain toxic waste sites have reduced some of the worst contamination. A 1987 U.S. Geological Survey report on water quality trends found that since federal water legislation was enacted, the nation's rivers showed a reduced fecal bacterial count, indicating better sewage treatment; a decline in lead concentrations; and higher levels of dissolved oxygen, suggesting a decrease in waterborne nutrients, primarily phosphates from laundry detergents, and nitrates from farm runoff, sewage plants, and industrial emissions. It is again possible to swim at many formerly closed beaches. Fish can now survive in waters that were once too polluted to support marine life.

In addition, water departments from Boston to San Francisco have begun to plug leaks in distribution systems, put locks on fire hydrants, and encourage customers to reduce water consumption. Improved efficiency in irrigation and other water conservation measures are helping to quench the growing national thirst for drinking water. With the price of new water supplies likely to skyrocket over the next two decades, these trends are certain to continue.

The Long Road Ahead

Unfortunately, the objective of the Clean Water Act and related regulations—pure surface water—is still far from being realized. The fish that have returned to the revitalized waters are often so full of dangerous chemicals that anglers are warned to eat them sparingly or not at all. Hundreds of toxic chemicals are still routinely found in the nation's rivers. A few alarming stories illustrate the grave problems that remain:

- Almost 2,000 industrial concerns have permits to discharge wastes into the Ohio River. More than twenty cities return treated sewage into the Ohio, and take their drinking water from the same source. Hundreds of synthetic chemicals are found in water samples drawn from the river.
- Every day, more than 100 tons of toxic chemicals are carried past New Orleans by the Mississippi River, the source of the city's drinking water. Nobody knows for sure how many of these substances travel unscathed through water treatment plants and are distributed into the city's water system, nor what their cumulative health effects are. What is known is that the residents of New Orleans have one of the nation's highest rates of cancer. A coincidence? It seems unlikely.
- In 1989, the EPA collected data on twelve million acres of lakes in thirty-four states. According to the agency's report, water quality is impaired in 25 percent of the surveyed lakes and threatened in another 20 percent. Seventy-five percent of the pollution comes from agricultural and urban runoff, with another 11 percent from industrial or sewage effluent.

Drinking water drawn from such polluted sources requires purification that is beyond the capabilities of most water treatment plants. While plants can effectively remove biological pathogens, they are simply not equipped to deal with a chemical cornucopia of such dimensions. Worse, chemical interactions at drinking water treatment plants can transform certain compounds to more dangerous contaminants, so the concentration of certain toxic substances is actually increased.

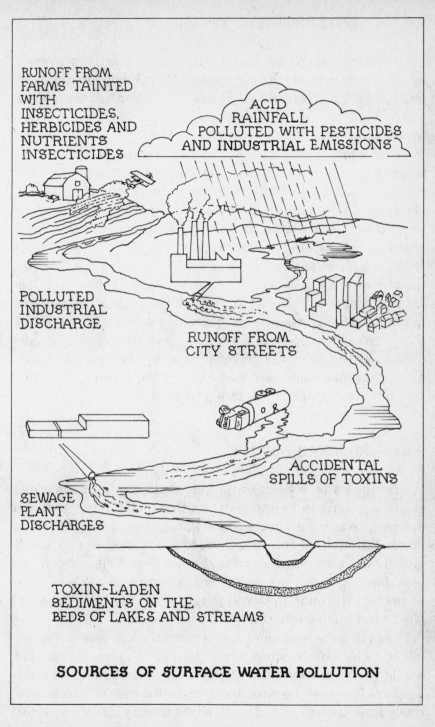

RUNOFF FROM FARMS TAINTED WITH INSECTICIDES, HERBICIDES AND NUTRIENTS INSECTICIDES

ACID RAINFALL POLLUTED WITH PESTICIDES AND INDUSTRIAL EMISSIONS

POLLUTED INDUSTRIAL DISCHARGE

RUNOFF FROM CITY STREETS

ACCIDENTAL SPILLS OF TOXINS

SEWAGE PLANT DISCHARGES

TOXIN-LADEN SEDIMENTS ON THE BEDS OF LAKES AND STREAMS

SOURCES OF SURFACE WATER POLLUTION

It will take scientists decades to analyze the danger posed by the chemicals in surface water and to devise methods of dealing with it. Until then, we can do little more than speculate about how toxic chemicals interact in a given water source and what their health effects are.

Meanwhile, other sources of surface water pollution continue to pose new hazards. Acid rain is the most publicized example. Thanks in large measure to emissions from power plants and automobiles, rainwater in the Northeast is five times as acidic as that in similar regions in undeveloped parts of the world. Rainfall in New York's Catskill Mountains is ten to twenty times as acidic as normal. According to a 1986 National Academy of Sciences report, this tainted rainfall has led to a dramatic increase in the acidity of lakes and streams in much of the Northeast and parts of the West over the last fifty years. The deterioration of statues and other stone formations is the most visible result, but acidic water also corrodes water-handling facilities, making the water that passes through more prone to contamination.

POLLUTED GROUNDWATER

Groundwater collects in porous underground formations called aquifers and supplies the other half of the nation's domestic water supply. Groundwater, which originates as precipitation, fills the spaces between the layers of sand, gravel, and rocks that make up an aquifer. Wells, which tap into these aquifers, supply at least a portion of the water for 75 percent of community water systems in the United States. Most rural homes rely solely on groundwater.

Until about a decade ago, groundwater was commonly believed to be safe because it was thought that rocks and soil would filter out toxic substances before they could reach the aquifer. For that reason, most groundwater receives relatively little treatment before it makes its way into your home.

But in the 1970s, pesticides and nitrates were detected in wells throughout agricultural regions and that assumption was shattered. Recent research, in fact, has found that groundwater is actually more vulnerable to pollution than surface water. Worse, the contamination is much harder to analyze and clean up. Some other surprises have turned up as well:

- Volatile chemicals that readily evaporate aboveground can accumulate to alarmingly high levels when denied access to the natural cleansing action of wind and sun. The solvent trichloroethylene (TCE), for instance, has been measured in groundwater at concentrations 2,000 times greater than any found in surface water. A sample taken from an aquifer under a Martin Marietta guided missile plant southwest of Denver contained 300,000 parts per billion (ppb) TCE; the highest level ever recorded in a river is 160 ppb. TCE is a suspected human carcinogen that has caused stomach and liver cancer and birth defects in animal tests.
- Aquifer contamination can go undetected for many years. In 1950, an aquifer under the village of Norwich, England, was found to be contaminated with whale oil, which had not been processed in the region since 1815. Eventually, an aquifer can become so soaked with poisonous compounds that it is difficult, if not impossible, to restore.
- Even when its source is known, mapping the spread of pollution in an aquifer is difficult and costs millions of dollars. Several monitoring wells and months of expensive consulting work are sometimes required to determine the speed and pattern of groundwater flow, which can be as much as several feet per day or as little as several inches per year.
- Stopping a plume of pollution can be expensive. The most effective techniques—building subterranean barriers to curtail the movement of contaminated water

and removing polluted water from an aquifer so that it can be treated—are even more costly than pollution mapping.

Sources of Pollution

We now know that groundwater pollution has myriad sources and can be found just about anywhere. Petroleum products, radioactive materials, and industrial solvents are just part of the toxic burden carried by the nation's groundwater. Leaky landfills, agricultural irrigation and pesticides, and polluted surface water are other common and hazardous sources of pollution. Faulty septic tanks, solvents from household cleaners and degreasers, septic tank cleaners, and nutrients from detergents and sewage all release diffuse, but highly toxic, contaminants into the water as well.

LUST: Leaking underground storage tanks (known by the spicy acronym LUST) are one of the most pervasive sources of groundwater contamination. There are almost five million buried tanks in the United States that contain substances considered too hazardous to store above ground, including liquid fuels, pesticides, industrial chemicals, and toxic wastes. About half of these tanks contain gas.

Corroded or cracked tanks, bad piping connections, and accidents have allowed toxic substances to seep into aquifers literally everywhere storage tanks are buried. Five percent of underground gasoline tanks are leaking, according to estimates by the EPA and the American Petroleum Institute, causing as much as 40 percent of the nation's groundwater pollution. Many abandoned storage tanks have been discovered only after nearby wells are found to be contaminated with gasoline or other toxic chemicals.

Here's a typical story about the origins and consequences of LUST. One summer day in 1988, an attendant at the Berkshire Marathon gas station in Crystal Park, Illinois, opened the access door to an underground gas tank and dropped in a wooden measuring stick. The stick plunged to the bottom with too much force, poking a hole about the size of a quarter in the bottom of the fiberglass tank. Before the ensuing leak was discovered, an estimated 7,000 gallons of premium unleaded gas had spewed into the underlying aquifer. Six months later, more than $100,000 had been spent cleaning up and assessing the damage caused by the leak. State officials predict it will cost $500,000 to remove the gasoline from the aquifer under the station, which is located 250 feet from a public water well.

Even a small gasoline leak can cause large problems. One gallon of gas seeping each day into an aquifer can poison a water supply used by hundreds of thousands of people. Yet because the tank's owner is unlikely to notice such a loss, small leaks can continue for long periods of time. A sensitive nose will detect gasoline in water at a concentration of one part per billion, which is about the smallest concentration modern testing equipment can reliably detect. Susceptible individuals may become ill when just a few parts of gas are diluted in a billion parts of drinking water.

In an effort to curb the flow of contamination, Congress passed amendments to the Resource Conservation Recovery Act in 1984 that imposed stiff new requirements on the owners of underground storage tanks. Among the mandates of the legislation are the installation of leak-detection equipment, the replacement of faulty tanks, and the purchase of liability insurance to cover aquifer cleanup costs in the event of a leak. The EPA predicts that owners of gasoline tanks eventually will have to spend $50 billion to comply with the new standards and that about one-third of the nation's small filling stations will go out of business because of associated costs.

INJECTION WELLS: Injection wells, another source of groundwater pollution, are essentially wells that run in reverse—pumps inject hazardous materials into formations believed capable of isolating them, often thousands of feet

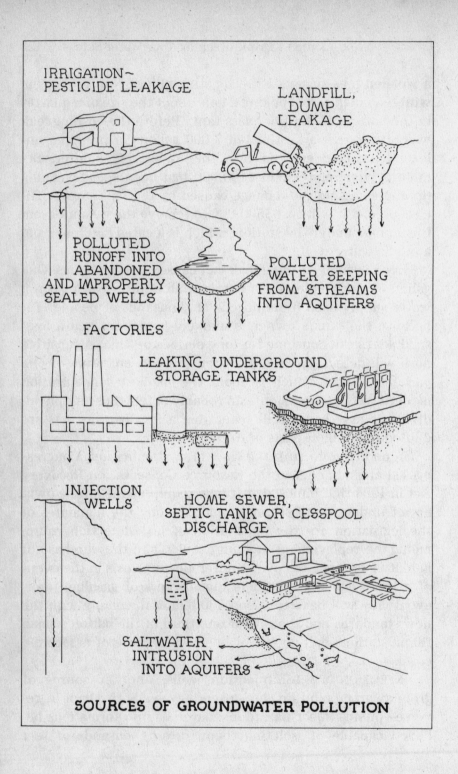

SOURCES OF GROUNDWATER POLLUTION

below the ground's surface. As surface disposal of toxic wastes grows more expensive, these wells have become increasingly popular, but the unexpected flow pattern of underground water has sometimes made it impossible to use them. Also, some injection wells have been abandoned when the chemicals ate their way through the rocks within which they were stored. The result, in either case, is severely contaminated groundwater.

CONTAMINATION IN THE TREATMENT AND DISTRIBUTION PROCESS

Water en route to the faucets of American homes and workplaces travels through a maze of reservoirs, tunnels, canals, aqueducts, pumping stations, treatment facilities, and water mains. Surface water used by community water systems, especially those located in arid regions, may flow through hundreds of miles of pipelines to reach its destination. Groundwater, on the other hand, is usually pumped into local wells and travels just a few miles to reach the water tap.

Like so many other components of the infrastructure, the average U.S. water system is in poor shape. Typically, pipes and pipelines are old and worn. Water, the "universal solvent," breaks down and absorbs a wide range of toxins present in many components of the aging system. A hole in pipe can also become a pathway by which contaminants from the soil can penetrate the distribution system. The growing acidity of rainwater in many regions further accelerates the aging of water-handling facilities because acidic water is aggressive, or corrosive.

Regions with soft water, which carries relatively few minerals, are more susceptible to contamination in the treatment and distribution process than hard water, which coats the inside of pipes and valves with a layer of minerals, protecting them from corrosion. Because it is already carrying a heavy

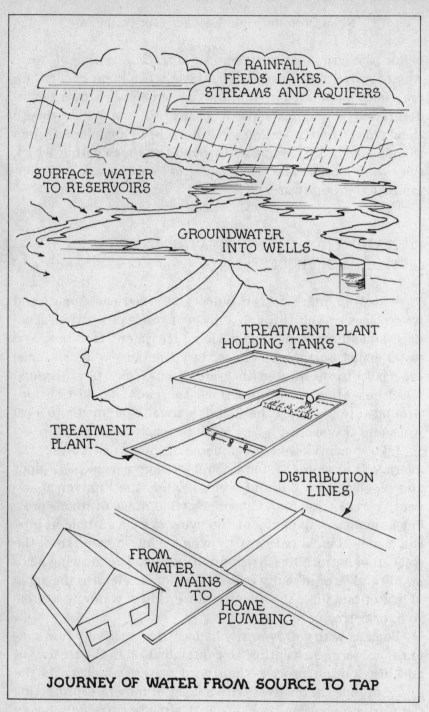

JOURNEY OF WATER FROM SOURCE TO TAP

load of minerals, hard water is also limited in its ability to pick up additional contaminants. Unfortunately, the mineral coating reduces a pipe's carrying capacity and can eventually lead to a sort of "hardening of the arteries," where the flow of water becomes so restricted by mineral buildup that the piping must be replaced.

The twin tunnels that siphon water from the Catskills and the headwaters of the Delaware River to New York City are among the relics threatened by the increasing acidity of surface water and the demands of a huge metropolis. Although the city has long enjoyed a reputation for top-notch drinking water, these tunnels haven't been shut down for inspection since they were put into service in the early part of the century because alone neither has sufficient capacity to meet the city's demand for water and no backup system exists.

The increasing acidity of the billion-and-a-half gallons of water that pass through the tunnels each day is undoubtedly accelerating their decay. Just how serious the problem is won't be known until the year 2000, when the thirteen-mile first phase of a new water tunnel, now being bored through bedrock 200 to 800 feet underground, is completed. The rest of the sixty-mile tunnel system is slated for completion by 2020, at a cost of $5 billion. The hope of New Yorkers, of course, is that the system will hold together until then.

Here is a look at the current process by which drinking water travels from its source into our homes.

The Treatment Process

After it has been transported from its source to a local water system, most surface water must be processed in a treatment plant before it can be used. Some groundwater, on the other hand, is considered chemically and biologically pure enough to pass directly from a well into the distribution system that carries it to the home.

Although there are innumerable variations, surface water

is usually treated as follows: First, it enters a storage lagoon where a chemical, usually copper sulfate, is added to control algae growth. From there, water passes through one or more screens that remove large debris. Next, a coagulant, such as alum, is mixed into the water to encourage the settling of suspended particles. The water flows slowly through one or more sedimentation basins so that larger particles settle to the bottom and can be removed. Water then passes through a filtration basin partially filled with sand and gravel where yet more suspended particles are removed.

At this point in the process, the Safe Drinking Water Act has mandated an additional step for communities using surface water. By 1991, water is to be filtered through activated carbon to remove any microscopic organic material and chemicals that have escaped the other processes. Activated carbon is extremely porous—one pound of the material can have a surface area of one acre. This honeycomb of minute pores attracts and traps pollutants through a process called adsorption.

Most water utilities, however, are seeking exemptions from the legislation on the grounds that it is too expensive. The estimated costs of installing activated carbon filtration in a water system designed to serve 50,000 people is about $4 million. A filtration plant capable of cleaning all the water for a major metropolitan area can easily cost billions of dollars. All told, American water utilities will have to spend an average of $5 billion to $10 billion per year to keep pace with the new standards, according to EPA estimates.

The final stage of water treatment is disinfection, where an agent capable of killing most biological pathogens is added to the water. Until the chlorination process was developed, devastating epidemics—such as the outbreak of typhoid and cholera that took 90,000 lives in Chicago in 1885—once spread wildly through community water systems. By 1910, most large water utilities had begun to chlorinate their surface water, and chlorine gas remains the disinfectant most widely used among community water systems.

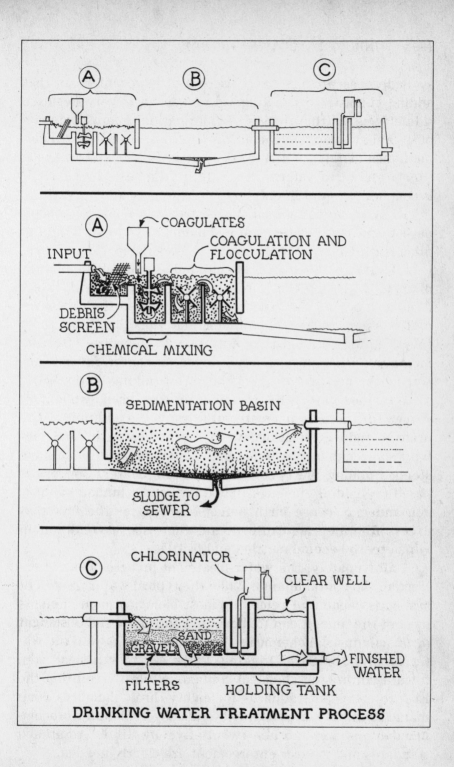

A COAGULATES
COAGULATION AND FLOCCULATION
INPUT
DEBRIS SCREEN
CHEMICAL MIXING

B SEDIMENTATION BASIN
SLUDGE TO SEWER

C CHLORINATOR
CLEAR WELL
GRAVEL SAND
FILTERS
HOLDING TANK
FINSHED WATER

DRINKING WATER TREATMENT PROCESS

Sadly, researchers have discovered in recent years that adding chlorine to drinking water has some very negative side effects. In the process of chlorination, microscopic bits of organic matter are chemically altered to produce trihalomethanes (THMs), a family of chemicals believed to cause cancer and birth defects. Chloroform, the best-known THM, is commonly found in chlorinated drinking water.

To meet the EPA limit of 100 parts of THMs per billion parts of drinking water, many communities are switching to other disinfectants with fewer objectionable side effects. Ozone, chlorine dioxide, and chloramine (which is a mixture of ammonia and chlorine) are among the alternative disinfectants now being used. Another way to prevent the formation of THMs is to remove the organic materials that allow them to form. Activated carbon filtration is the most effective method to accomplish this, a strong argument in favor of enforcing the new mandates of the Safe Drinking Water Act.

A further step in the treatment process, used by about 60 percent of the nation's water utilities, is the addition of fluoride to reduce tooth decay. In recent years, this has met with some public resistance and a number of utilities have stopped adding the chemical to drinking water. Concern is based on limited evidence that fluoride is a human carcinogen and may cause birth defects, as well as the fact that excess fluoride can cause dental fluorosis, a condition in which teeth become mottled and brittle.

Unfortunately, the water treatment process does not extract all the contaminants. While the typical water treatment system is capable of removing most biological contaminants most of the time, it cannot begin to control the full onslaught of toxic industrial chemicals that find their way into the water supply. The Safe Drinking Water Act took a small step toward controlling chemical contamination by requiring the EPA to establish standards for eighty-three chemicals commonly found in water supply systems by 1989 and to recommend limits for another twenty-five by 1991. Additional standards and greater enforcement are clearly needed.

The Distribution System

Once it leaves the treatment plant, water can pick up additional toxic substances as it flows through a network of distribution pipes to your home. Pipe corrosion and chemical reactions allow lead, cadmium, asbestos, vinyl chloride, THMs, and numerous other contaminants to enter the water. Leaky pipes, which allow as much as one-third of the treated water to be lost, also permit additional impurities to enter the system, especially when it is shut down for repairs. Bacterial growths and corrosion can further contaminate water, and ironically, so can the herbicides and anticorrosion agents employed to control them.

The materials used in pipes themselves are further sources of contamination. More than 200,000 miles of asbestos-cement water supply pipes are in use in the United States. Although asbestos-cement pipe is marketed as being immune to corrosion, aggressive water can attack it and allow the asbestos fibers to be released into the water. A 1979 EPA study found that in 20 percent of the surveyed cities, water carried more than one million fibers of asbestos per liter—11 percent had more than ten million fibers per liter.

Plastic water mains are becoming more common because of demonstrated resistance to corrosion, low cost, and ease of installation and repair. Unfortunately, vinyl chloride, a known human carcinogen, is a primary ingredient of plastic pipes. Vinyl chloride, as well as heavy metals, which are added to increase the pipe's resistance to heat, can leech into the water. Making matters worse, toxic compounds, including dimethylformamide (DMF), a suspected carcinogen, are employed in the primers and solvent cements used to fasten the pipes together. A further problem is that THMs can form when impurities in the water react with the components of plastic piping. And if water mains pass through contaminated ground, as many do, gasoline components and other toxic substances can penetrate plastic pipe and cause contamination.

If you live in a rural area with a private well, the source of your water is much closer to home—probably no more than a few hundred feet away. Even in this short journey, however, there is ample opportunity for contamination. Long lengths of plastic pipe often snake from the well to the aquifer, and if the plastic is deteriorating, chemicals may leach into the water. Biological contaminants are troublesome in rural wells.

Domestic Plumbing

If your drinking water manages to complete the expedition from its source to your home relatively unscathed by pollution, there is only one further barrier to its pristine emergence from your kitchen tap: the building's plumbing system. Lead, which was commonly used in the plumbing systems of homes, schools, and office buildings until the 1930s, and in solder to fasten copper piping until 1986, is one of the biggest dangers. Officials in Washington, D.C., conducted a survey in 1987 and found that tap water in at least 71,000 of the city's homes contained unsafe concentrations of lead that could be traced to residential plumbing. And in Chicago it was actually illegal until recently to connect household plumbing to city water mains with anything but lead piping. (That quirky regulation can be traced to the power of the plumber's union, whose members earned a healthy income by making the required hookup for residents.) Now it will cost an estimated $1.5 billion to replace those lead connecting pipes.

Here's what happened at an EPA building at the Federal Plaza complex in lower Manhattan in 1985: After employees complained of a metallic taste in the water fountains, investigators analyzed the water and discovered that lead levels registered 200 parts per billion—ten times the current EPA threshold for community water systems. Bottled water had to be provided throughout the building, at a cost of $35,000 per month, until the source of the problem could be traced. Eventually, a lead pipe that connected the building's water system to city water mains, coupled with lead solder in the building's plumbing, were identified as the villains. Once the lead pipe was replaced with stainless steel, the problem vanished.

Zinc, organic chemicals, and biological growths can also taint the water as it passes through household pipes. Unfortunately, these and other substances can accumulate in the hot water heater and pose a threat even when filtering systems are used. Another often-overlooked danger is plastic pipe, which California banned for use in home plumbing systems in 1980 because of the associated health risks.

Whatever the source of the contamination, ordinary household activities can transfer many of the toxins found in your water to indoor air. Agitating water—by boiling it on the stove, spraying it from a kitchen tap, shower head, or bathtub faucet, or swishing it around in a washing machine—speeds the evaporation of dissolved toxic substances. Heating also reduces the ability of a gas to remain in solution, so contaminants are particularly likely to be released when the hot water tap is on. Radon, benzene, and chloroform are among the dissolved gases that easily evaporate into indoor air, where they can be inhaled.

Contaminants can also enter the body through the skin. For example, a fifty-pound child spending an hour splashing in a pool or a bathtub filled with polluted water can absorb ten times more toxic substances than drinking a quart of the same water. Higher water temperatures, breaks in the skin, rashes, and sunburn all increase the rate at which these substances pass into the body.

THE CONTAMINANTS

Here's a closer look at some of the contaminants routinely found in drinking water:

Gasoline Components
- Benzene: Benzene compounds are among the most toxic

of the 250 or more chemicals contained in gasoline. While the EPA took action in August 1989 to limit the benzene content of gasoline, the potent carcinogen continues to be in solvents, plastics, paint removers, and other popular household products. Benzene is extremely volatile and easily evaporates from water, creating both air and water pollution problems.

- Ethylene dibromide (EDB): EDB was developed by Dow Chemical Company in the 1920s as a gasoline additive to help remove lead from internal combustion engines. From the 1940s to the 1980s, EDB was also widely used as an insecticide. Because of its extreme toxicity, its use is now heavily restricted, but the chemical continues to be found in groundwater.

Radioactive Materials

- Radium: A decay product of uranium found primarily in groundwater, the highest concentrations of radium have been measured in Iowa, Illinois, Wisconsin, and Missouri.
- Radon: The EPA estimates that as much as half the radon found in the air of homes in the northeastern United States has evaporated from groundwater.
- Uranium: This contaminant is found primarily in aquifers composed of granitic gravel. Uranium in surface water is primarily a problem in the western states and comes almost entirely from piles of waste rock at uranium mines and in the wastes created by the smelting process.

Industrial Chemicals

- Dioxin: Dioxins are found as impurities in herbicides (most notoriously in Agent Orange, the defoliant used in Vietnam), and in pentachlorophenol, a wood preservative. In 1983, dioxin contamination converted most of Times Beach, Missouri, a community of 2,200 located southwest of St. Louis, into a ghost town. Local soil and groundwater became contaminated after waste oil con-

taining dioxin was spread on roads and parking lots and used for dust control on local farms.
- Polychlorinated biphenols: PCBs are a family of more than 200 carcinogenic chemicals used primarily in electrical equipment. The lower Hudson River in New York has some of the highest concentrations in the nation, the result of decades of waste dumping by General Electric and other plants in New York City and New Jersey. PCB-bearing sediments on the river's bed will continue to pollute the Hudson's water for decades.
- Trichloroethylene (TCE): This solvent, the active ingredient of many septic tank cleaners and industrial degreasers, has been found in aquifers in every part of the country.

Pesticides
- Aldicarb: Produced by Union Carbide under the trade name Temik, aldicarb is used to control insects on potatoes, peanuts, sugar beets, citrus crops, and cotton. It has been found in groundwater in all parts of the country, with especially high concentrations on Long Island, New York. Aldicarb has been banned in twelve states but is not regulated nationally.
- Alachlor: The most widely used herbicide in the country, alachlor kills weeds found with corn, soybeans, and other crops. It is produced by Monsanto under the trade name Lasso. This potent animal carcinogen has been found in groundwater in most parts of the nation.

Heavy Metals
- Lead: Water that passes through lead pipes or comes in contact with lead solder can easily become contaminated, as we've already discussed. Runoff from city streets, which is usually tainted with lead from automobile exhaust and spilled gasoline, leaking gasoline storage tanks, mine and mill tailings, and junked batteries are other common sources of lead pollution in both surface and groundwater. Lead-lined water cool-

ers remain in widespread use, although they were banned in 1988. The high lead content in the drinking water of many schools has contributed to a nationwide increase in the average lead concentration in children's blood. Brain damage, hearing impairments, and hindered nervous-system development are the tragic results.

- Cadmium: Cadmium leaches into the drinking water from corroded galvanized steel pipes and from plastic pipes. Mines, smelters, and the electroplating industry also commonly pollute lakes, streams, and aquifers with the suspected carcinogen.
- Arsenic: Runoff from the tailings of mines and smelters, as well as wastes produced by pesticide manufacturers, often pollute streams with this toxic metal. Arsenic emitted from the smokestacks of smelters and some industries also finds its way into both surface and groundwater.
- Mercury: One of the least abundant elements in the Earth's crust, this metal is associated with paper-mill wastes and the manufacture of electrical equipment. Mercury was also used in the production of nuclear weapons until the mid-1960s. Although it has been more than twenty years since the metal was used at the Department of Energy's nuclear weapons facilities at Oak Ridge, Tennessee, the underlying aquifer at the site remains so saturated with mercury that an estimated two ounces oozes into a nearby creek every day.

Toxic Substances from the Water System

- Asbestos: The asbestos-cement water pipe used in many distribution systems is responsible for most of the asbestos found in drinking water. Ore-processing plants, asbestos-cement roofing tile, and siding can also spew asbestos fibers into lakes and streams.
- Methylene chloride: Methylene chloride, a volatile organic compound used in the production of paints, in-

secticides, solvents, and many other products, often contaminates lakes, streams, and aquifers. Water utilities were required to start monitoring for methylene chloride in 1989.

- Phthalates: This class of organic chemicals is widely employed in the production of plastics. DEHP, one of the most common phthalates, constitutes some 40 percent of the mass of polyvinyl chloride pipe. Water bottled in plastic containers and drinking water that has passed through plastic pipe often contain DEHP and other phthalates.
- Vinyl chloride: This carcinogen leaches into drinking water primarily from polyvinyl chloride pipe. Water that stands in pipes overnight or longer is most contaminated.
- Trihalomethanes (THMs): Chloroform, bromochloromethane, bromodichloromethane, and bromoform are formed when impurities in the water supply react with chlorine and with the components of plastic water pipe.

Biological Agents
- Coliform bacteria: Fecal coliform bacteria come from human and animal waste. They are not toxic, but their presence in a water sample indicates that harder-to-detect and potentially more virulent organisms may also be present.
- Giardia cysts: Giardia cysts, the larval form of a parasite deposited into the water primarily from the feces of beaver and other water animals, thrive in cold mountain streams. One beaver can put more than one million cysts per day into the water, contaminating remote watersheds that are otherwise pure. When ingested by a human, the giardia parasite can attach itself to the wall of the intestines, drawing nutrients from the stream of partially digested food passing by. As it multiplies, the parasite can cause a lingering, flulike malady characterized by diarrhea. Because the para-

sites can survive in chlorinated water, some community water systems have installed activated carbon filters to remove giardia cysts.

SOLUTIONS: HOW TO CLEAN UP YOUR DRINKING WATER

Step One: Learn and Conserve

Because a wise consumer is an educated one, the best place to start your battle for clean drinking water is by learning more about water quality problems in your community. Some sources for additional information:

- The local water utility, which is required to test for contaminants regulated under the Safe Drinking Water Act. A summary of results is generally available on request.
- The local health department, which usually tracks the presence of contaminants and minerals in the water.
- Local citizen-action organizations that are lobbying to clean up the water.
- The index of your local newspaper, available in most public libraries, may help you identify polluters in the area and alert you to past problems.
- National hotlines, from which you can learn more about water quality and programs designed to safeguard it.

A related step is to make a commitment to water conservation. Although water is a renewable resource, it is not one to be squandered thoughtlessly. Along with making a tangible contribution to the environmental health of your community, reducing water consumption has a direct impact on your pocketbook. If you filter all your household water, as we recommend in the following pages, conservation efforts mean you have less water to treat so the filter doesn't need to be replaced as often. By reducing hot water use, you'll also save on gas and electricity costs. Since the price of both water and energy is certain to increase dramatically over the next decade, it makes good sense to begin conservation efforts now.

An alternative to filtration is to drink only bottled water. A 1989 survey of customers of the Los Angeles Metropolitan Water Department found that 53 percent used bottled water and another 19 percent filter their tap water because they don't like the water's chemical taste or are concerned about health effects. Pesticides, industrial solvents, and salts are routinely found in the Los Angeles water system, which is supplied by the Colorado River and reservoirs in the Sierra Nevada Mountains. Bottled water is widely available and generally of good quality, although it costs more than filtered water and is not a solution to the problems associated with volatile chemicals in the shower or bathtub.

Step Two: Test Your Water

Before you can decide how to improve the drinking water in your home, you'll need to know just what's wrong with it. While some toxic substances are difficult to detect even with sophisticated equipment a good test can measure most of the more common ones. The equipment and analysis generally costs about $100, although some laboratories offer special rates for first-time customers.

Testing equipment is available from the national testing laboratories listed in the Appendix, or you may find local labs in your telephone book. Some companies that market water purification devices offer a free water test, but remember: They have a product to sell and therefore have a motive to exaggerate the seriousness of test results. Your local health department may also offer free testing for biological contaminants.

To obtain a reliable picture of the contents of your water, you'll need to perform two or more tests at different times of the year, since seasonal variations in the level of surface and groundwater can affect its quality. The lab will provide you with specimen bottles and instructions for collecting samples. Usually, you will be instructed to sterilize your faucets and to run the tap for a few minutes in order to purge any standing water before filling the bottles. Be sure to follow the lab's instructions to the letter to ensure valid test results.

After analyzing your water sample, the company will send a report that describes its findings and alerts you to the presence of any contaminants at higher-than-recommended levels. Some labs will also advise you about how to remove the contaminants.

Another part of the diagnostic process is a measure of the acidity (pH) and hardness of your water. That information is generally collected by the water utility. If the pH is more than 7 or the hardness is less than 60, the water may be corroding your pipes, picking up additional contaminants in the process.

If your plumbing system is more than fifty years old, it is also important to inspect the pipes for the presence of lead. The exterior surface of lead pipes is a dull gray; when scraped with a pocketknife, the coating is easily removed to reveal a shiny surface. Lead-soldered copper piping can be identified by the dull gray metal around the joints. If there are brass fittings at the joints, it is unlikely that there is lead solder in the system.

Step Three: Choose a Water Purification System

If lab results indicate that your water has contamination problems, you will have to choose a purification system that best meets your needs. Most people opt to filter only their drinking water, but ideally, you should filter all the water in your house to reduce the contaminants released into the air from the shower, bathtub, spa, washing machine, and dishwasher. If toxic volatile chemicals (such as TCE, benzene, and radon) are present, whole-house filtration is definitely appropriate.

Eliminating lead contamination from a home plumbing system cannot be done solely with filtration, although a point-of-use filter on the kitchen tap can help. Ideally, lead-soldered copper plumbing should be replaced, but this can cost more than $1,000. A less costly and fairly effective solution to minimize your lead exposure is to run the water for a few minutes before using it for cooking or drinking.

Three basic types of water purification systems are commonly available:

• *Activated carbon filters* are the most effective means of removing many of the very small, but extremely toxic, substances found in water. They are also the most practical way to purify all the water in a residence. With an activated carbon filter, water passes through either granules or a solid

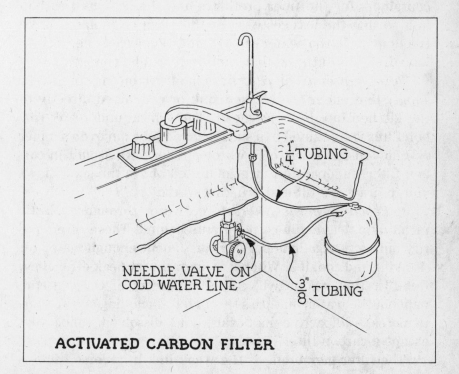

ACTIVATED CARBON FILTER

block of specially prepared carbon. Powdered carbon should be avoided since it can mix with water and redeposit filtered contaminants.

The effectiveness of an activated carbon filter depends on the amount of time water is exposed to the carbon (the longer the better), the manner in which the water flows through the filter medium (the more diffuse its path, the better), and the number and size range of the micropores in the carbon (the greater the range, the more contaminants that can be removed).

Activated carbon filters come in a variety of configurations. *Whole-house filters* are mounted on the house's main water supply line and usually require a plumber's expertise. Water passes first through one or more fiber prefilters, which remove larger contaminants, then through the carbon element. The best whole-house filtering systems use separate containers for the fiber prefilters and the activated carbon unit so that the less costly fiber filter can be replaced more frequently. If the water supply line is inaccessible, it may have to be rerouted so that the filters can be changed.

Point-of-use carbon filters are mounted on the cold water supply line under the kitchen sink or connected directly to the kitchen tap or showerhead. The typical under-sink carbon filter is contained in a single plastic tube; an even simpler system consists solely of a water pitcher with a built-in carbon filter. A separate faucet mounted above the sink allows you to draw the filtered drinking water.

• *Reverse-osmosis filters* force water through a plastic membrane, leaving most pollutants behind. These filters purify only a few gallons per day, just about enough water for drinking and cooking. When it is operating at peak efficiency, this filtration system will catch 90 percent of the contaminants in the water that pass through it, including certain particulates, radioactive materials, and dissolved solids that escape a carbon filter.

The filter membrane is the weak link in reverse osmosis

filtration. Some won't filter chlorinated water unless a carbon filter is first used to remove the chlorine. Others quickly become clogged with bacterial growth if the water is not chlorinated. The membrane may also miss some of the very smallest toxins that can be adsorbed by a carbon filter.

The best reverse-osmosis filtration systems employ three

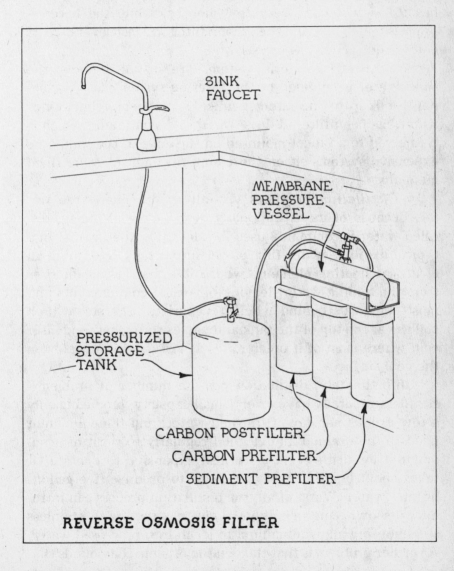

SINK
FAUCET

MEMBRANE
PRESSURE
VESSEL

PRESSURIZED
STORAGE
TANK

CARBON POSTFILTER
CARBON PREFILTER
SEDIMENT PREFILTER

REVERSE OSMOSIS FILTER

filtration steps using three separate containers. Ideally, a particulate prefilter first strains out sediment, then a reverse-osmosis filter removes some of the smaller dissolved materials and larger organic chemicals; and finally, activated carbon filters out volatile organic chemicals and other microscopic contaminants. In this sort of system, the prefilter typically has to be replaced every few months, while the reverse-osmosis membrane and the carbon filter will last several years before replacement is necessary.

Some reverse-osmosis systems are installed under the sink. Water is supplied to the filtering system via a permanent hookup to the kitchen faucet's cold water line. Once water has been filtered, it is stored in a small tank, which is connected to a faucet mounted on the edge of the sink. Less expensive systems sit on the countertop and must be filled manually.

• *Distillation* produces virtually contaminant-free water. Because of its exceptionally high degree of purity, distilled water is commonly used in scientific experiments. In a typical distiller, water first passes into a tank containing an electrical heating element, where it is boiled. Steam rises from the boiling water, leaving biological contaminants and most chemicals behind when it vaporizes. The steam then collects at the top of the tank and passes through a condenser coil, where most of it precipitates as virtually pure water on the cool surfaces.

Unfortunately, distillation poses a number of problems. Distillers generally have a very small capacity, producing only a few gallons per day of finished water, and the equipment needs to be drained and cleaned regularly to rid it of accumulated impurities. They are also expensive to operate—it takes about one dollar of electricity to produce five gallons of pure water. Worst of all, the distillation process can introduce its own contamination. Some distillers with stainless steel housing allow aluminum to leach into processed water. A further problem is that the volatile organic compounds that evaporate as the water is heated can be drawn off the top of the boiling tank with the steam and pass into finished water in the condenser coil.

To avoid this problem, some manufacturers have added an activated carbon filter to remove the chemicals or a valve at the top of the boiling chamber that vents volatiles before they pass into the condenser. Be sure to check for these features before making a purchase.

Smaller distillers are kept on the kitchen counter next to the sink. The least expensive units must be loaded by hand and turned on and off manually. More sophisticated products operate automatically; they are connected to the cold water supply line, which supplies water whenever the finished-water tank is drawn down. As with reverse-osmosis filters, the best distillation systems employ a fiber prefilter and a carbon postfilter to produce ultrapure water.

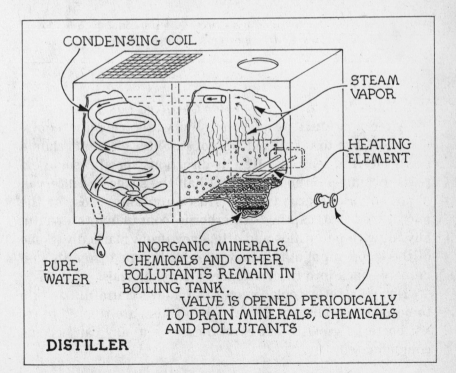

CONDENSING COIL

STEAM VAPOR

HEATING ELEMENT

PURE WATER

INORGANIC MINERALS, CHEMICALS AND OTHER POLLUTANTS REMAIN IN BOILING TANK.

VALVE IS OPENED PERIODICALLY TO DRAIN MINERALS, CHEMICALS AND POLLUTANTS

DISTILLER

Purchasing Water Purification Equipment

Before you commit to the purchase of water purification equipment, be certain you can answer the following questions:

- Do you want to filter all the water in your house or just the drinking water? What is the equipment's capacity?
- How much does the system cost?
- What guarantees are offered?
- How hard is it to install and use the purification equipment?
- How much will maintenance cost? How often must basic maintenance be performed?
- Are components that may taint finished water, such as plastic, used?

ADAPTED FROM: *But Not a Drop to Drink! The Life-Saving Guide to Good Water* by Steve Coffel (Rawson Associates, 1989).

Step Four: Maintain Your Water Cleaning Equipment

After you start using your new water cleaning equipment, be sure to take good care of it. Filter elements should be replaced at least as often as directions specify; some experts recommend replacement at half the suggested interval. If an activated carbon filter is used too long, most of the micropores that capture waterborne contaminants eventually fill with impurities and efficiency drops markedly. Some of the trapped pollutants may even be bumped from the micropores back into the water by other chemicals.

Delaying filter replacement also allows harmful bacteria to become established. Some carbon filters are treated to resist bacterial growth, but even these eventually can become contaminated.

If your drinking water is chlorinated, testing the effectiveness of a filter is easy. Commercially available kits will tell you whether chlorine is entering the finished water—if chlorine is passing through the filter, other toxic substances probably are as well. The filter should be promptly replaced.

It's a good idea to have your water tested annually, even after your purification equipment is installed. Think of it as insurance!

PART II:
AT WORK

7
ON THE JOB
Is Your Office Making
You Sick?

The conference room in a Westchester County, New York, office building is crowded with employees concerned about the problems of indoor air pollution. And for good reason. For three years now, workers have been complaining about stale air and disquieting health problems. And for three years investigators have searched for explanations—to no avail. This afternoon's meeting, one of a series being held throughout the county, begins with a twenty-minute slide show. Then the floor is opened for questions, comments, and complaints. No one holds back.

One worker described how long-standing health problems had been exacerbated in an environment where ventilation is inadequate. "I've got terrible allergies and they've worsened noticeably since I began working here," said a middle-aged man. "After the first week, I headed straight to the doctor for shots. The air is terribly stale here, and I can't draw a deep breath."

A high-level supervisor described the loss of productivity she had observed in her department. Her private office affords better air quality than the partitioned, windowless interior space where the clerical staff works and the executive noted, "When I step out from my office to talk with my secretary, I can immediately detect the poor air quality. And she's got to sit in that environment all day. I'm convinced that's why we're seeing a very noticeable drop in energy level as the day wears on."

One oft-repeated complaint was that cigarette smoke fouled the air and was slow to dissipate. Several participants expressed particular unhappiness that smokers and nonsmokers were permitted to work in close proximity to each other. "No one smokes in my immediate work area, but they smoke nearby and I can still smell the fumes," complained one woman. Another added, "Smokers leave our area for a cigarette, but when they return they exhale the smoke that collects in their lungs."

Despite assurances that their complaints would not fall on deaf ears, employees left the afternoon session with little conviction that indoor air quality problems would be resolved soon. "Those of us who have been here three or four years have been told 'We're working on the problem' too often to expect quick solutions," grumbled one worker. No single contaminant has been found to exceed permissible concentration levels in that Westchester County office building, and the source of its pollution problems remains a mystery. But no one is suggesting the problem doesn't exist; rather, the building is being cited as an example of the complexities involved in tracing the source of air quality problems in tightly sealed office buildings and implementing effective solutions.

Here are just a few other tales about buildings that make their inhabitants ill:

- In *The New York Times*, building in Manhattan's Times Square, birds found welcome nesting grounds near the air-conditioning equipment. Shortly after the birds settled in, two dozen employees became ill. The problem was eventually traced to fecal bacteria, which had entered the air conditioner and circulated through the building.
- In an elementary school on the outskirts of Washington, D.C., four teachers fell mysteriously ill and could not return to work for several months. Eventually, their devastating health problems were traced to the growth of mold on books and school materials. Because the building had been constructed on low-lying terrain without proper drainage, water had leaked through the

walls and caused a dampness that became an ideal breeding ground for biological organisms.

- In 1986 a faulty ventilation system at the veterinary school of the University of Florida in Gainesville forced faculty to abandon the structure while repairs were made. In the interim, $1 million of state funds were spent to purchase modular housing for the staff; another $3.4 million is being poured into an overhaul of the system.

Just what's happening at the workplace? Health hazards have long been associated with industrial processes and, tragic though it is, it is not surprising that factory workers are repeatedly exposed to high levels of toxic chemicals or that miners breathe poisoned air every time they descend into the pits. Painfully little attention has been paid to the occupational hazards of white-collar workers. Yet, many of the nation's sixty-five million office workers could be the innocent victims of perils we are just beginning to understand. In the short term, contaminants in the typical office building are more likely to cause a rash or the sniffles than a life-threatening disease. But not all symptoms are so innocuous—even a small amount of carbon monoxide, released into the air by cigarette smoke, can cause severe headaches, while the formaldehyde that outgasses from newly installed cabinetry has been linked to respiratory distress. The cumulative effect of low-level, long-term exposure to these and numerous other toxic substances is of great concern—all the more so, perhaps, because we have not yet determined just how grave the dangers truly are.

The leading villains of workplace pollution—faulty ventilation, chemical contamination, biological contamination, and asbestos—each deserve a closer look. First, though, it is important to look again at one of the root causes of the problem: the race to seal up office buildings in the name of energy conservation.

WHAT IS A SICK BUILDING?

The design and operation of commercial buildings were profoundly affected by the energy crisis of the 1970s. As fuel prices soared, developers and landlords became frantic to save on heating and air-conditioning costs. Engineers, architects, and builders responded by sealing costly air leaks wherever possible. As in the home, thermal doors and windows were installed, caulking and weather stripping became more widely used, and extra layers of insulation were blown into the ceilings, floors, and walls of older buildings. Operable windows, which reduce the efficiency of central heating and air-conditioning systems, were eliminated in most new construction.

The most significant cost-saving measures introduced directly in response to the energy crisis were adjustments in the heating, ventilation, and air-conditioning (HVAC) system. In addition to regulating room temperature and humidity levels, an HVAC system controls the amount of fresh air that is introduced into a building. To combat rising fuel costs, building owners upped the percentage of recirculated indoor air, which does not have to be artificially cooled or heated, while reducing the entry of outside air.

But now we appreciate the link between adequate ventilation and human health and comfort. We have discovered that bringing fresh air inside is the most effective way to rid the office of stale odors and the contaminants released from office equipment, building materials, furnishings, cigarette smoke, and elsewhere. And we have seen the consequences of barricading a building against fresh air.

Two terms have been coined to describe the problems that ensue: building-related illness (BRI) and sick building syndrome (SBS), also called tight building syndrome. *Building-related illnesses* are those in which well-identified diseases are traced to specific workplace problems. Typical building-related illnesses include hypersensitivity pneumonitis, humidifier fever, and Legionnaire's disease, all caused by microbial contamination. Skin irritations, caused by chemical-rich glues or solvents, are another example of BRI. Once the source of the symptoms is identified and eliminated, BRI generally disappears.

Often, though, it can be impossible to make such specific correlations. *Sick building syndrome* differs from building-related illnesses in that symptoms do not fit the pattern of one particular illness and cannot be clearly associated with a single cause. The syndrome usually occurs in a tightly sealed office building with inefficient or faulty ventilation and depends on a complex synergy among low levels of many contaminants. Symptoms can include dry or burning mucous membranes, eye, nose, and throat irritation, congestion, respiratory difficulties, lethargy, fatigue, irritability, headaches, dizziness, and difficulty with concentration.

Occasionally, sick building syndrome manifests itself in sudden and widespread illness and in a few extreme cases, buildings have been at least temporarily abandoned when contamination could not be traced or controlled. More often, evidence of a problem develops gradually. Absentee rates may climb, supervisors will report declining productivity, and employees begin to grumble about stuffiness, discomfort, or a range of health problems that subside after work and on the weekends. While these stories lack the drama of a disaster, they are a major drain on the economy, costing the nation untold billions of dollars in medical expenses and lost productivity. And the problem of sick building syndrome is growing; according to the World Health Organization, up to 30 percent of new or remodeled buildings have unusually high SBS complaints.

VENTILATION SYSTEMS: A TOOL FOR GOOD OR EVIL?

General ventilation and local ventilation are both necessary to move air through a building and to purge it of contaminants. General ventilation is provided through the HVAC system's buildingwide network of ducts, vents, fans, and coils, which also maintains room temperature at between 68°F and 75°F and relative humidity at a comfortable level between 35 and 60 percent (preferably between 30 and 50 percent in winter and between 40 and 60 percent in summer). Local exhaust ventilation is designed to capture toxic dust, fumes, and gas at their source and exhaust them outside. Although it is widely used in manufacturing processes that involve high concentrations of chemicals, the value of local ventilation is often overlooked in office buildings.

It's not necessary to become an engineering expert to understand the sources of workplace pollution, but a rudimentary understanding of mechanical ventilation certainly helps. Forearmed with some basic knowledge, employees can more readily make their own assessment of indoor air quality problems and lobby much more effectively for improvements.

An Engineering Primer: How HVAC Systems Work

An office building may be served by one or several HVAC systems. Even if one main system is used, additional perimeter units are often added to provide greater temperature control and sometimes to introduce additional fresh air. Inside air is a combination of fresh outside air (known as makeup air), which enters the building through intake vents, and recirculated indoor air. This blend travels through the HVAC system's network of supply ducts, passing through a series of air cleaners, which use filters to screen out dust particles, and charcoal beds, which reduce odor. Air-tempering units then regulate the temperature before a supply fan blows the air into occupied spaces through room vents. Depending on the type of HVAC system in use, the air may pass through a system of coils (also called a terminal unit), which is supplied with heating or cooling refrigerant that further regulates air temperature.

Stale air is exhausted from the room through a parallel

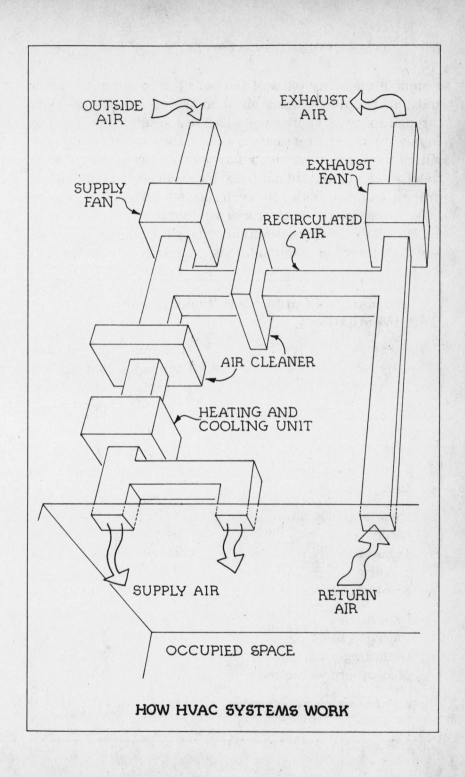

OUTSIDE AIR

EXHAUST AIR

SUPPLY FAN

EXHAUST FAN

RECIRCULATED AIR

AIR CLEANER

HEATING AND COOLING UNIT

SUPPLY AIR

RETURN AIR

OCCUPIED SPACE

HOW HVAC SYSTEMS WORK

system of ducts. An exhaust fan pulls the air out of the room and into the ducts; some air then travels out the building through exhaust vents, while the rest heads back into the supply ducts. The recirculated air is then cleaned and permitted to pass through the building again. Because very little fresh air can penetrate naturally into well-sealed buildings, a proper balance between recirculated air and fresh, or makeup, air is critical to proper ventilation.

Most HVAC systems simultaneously humidify the air, usually in winter, or dehumidify it, generally in summer, to

Recommended Outdoor Air Requirements for Ventilation

	Maximum Occupancy persons/ 1,000 feet	Ventilation Rates cf/m/ person*
Office Space		
Office	7	20
Conference room	50	20
Reception area	65	15
Educational Facilities		
Classroom	50	15
Laboratory	30	20
Library	20	15
Smoking lounge	70	60
Hospitals		
Patient's room	10	25
Operating room	20	30
Medical procedure room	20	15

*cubic feet per minute per person

maintain relative humidity at a comfortable level. Humidity is provided by spraying water or steam into the supply air-flow or allowing the air to pass through a tray of water or some other water-soaked media before it enters an occupied space. Air is generally dehumidified at the system cooling coils, where excess moisture condenses onto drain pans as air temperature drops.

According to the voluntary standards set by the American Society of Heating, Refrigeration and Air-conditioning Engineers, an efficient HVAC system will distribute fresh, out-

	Maximum Occupancy persons/ 1,000 feet	Ventilation Rates cf/m/ person*
Retail Spaces and Recreation		
Pharmacy	20	15
Supermarket	8	15
Beauty shop	25	25
Bowling alley	70	25
Ballroom and disco	100	25
Food and Beverage Services		
Restaurant dining room	70	20
Kitchen	20	15
Bar	100	30
Transportation		
Waiting room and platform	100	15
Vehicle	100	15

SOURCE: ASHRAE Standard 62-1989, "Ventilation for Acceptable Indoor Air Quality."

door air through an office building at a minimum rate of 15 cubic feet per minute (cf/m) per occupant. Ventilation requirements climb even higher for other building uses, as shown in the accompanying sidebar.

Local Exhaust Ventilation

Local exhaust ventilation, a necessary adjunct to an HVAC system, has the advantage of carrying off contaminants before they reach the breathing zone of most workers. Local, or spot, exhaust is used in building areas where a concentration of contaminants are generated by particular equipment or office processes; for example, good local ventilation is im-

---

Is the Local Ventilation System Working?

Answers to these questions will help determine whether design or operational flaws in the local exhaust ventilation system are contributing to indoor air quality problems:

1. Is the hood located as close as possible to the source of the contaminant?
2. Are filters clogged?
3. Is airflow into the hood adequate to capture air contaminants?
4. Are fumes, dust, or mist visibly drawn into the hood?
5. Is there any noticeable smell in the area of the hood?
6. Do workers notice any eye, nose, or throat irritation while the hood is running?
7. Are air contaminants pulled through the breathing zone of the worker?
8. Are ducts deteriorated or corroded? Are there holes or cracks in the ductwork?

portant to the safe use of photocopying or printing equipment, graphic arts materials, and solvents. By ridding a room of its most intensely concentrated pollutants at their source, spot exhaustion can lessen the ventilation demands placed on the HVAC system.

A local exhaust system consists of a hood that sucks in contaminated air, ducts that carry it away, and a collector or air-cleaning device that purifies the air before it is vented to the outside (to minimize outdoor pollution problems). One or more fans are used to move contaminated air out of the room and replace it with adequate makeup air.

A number of technical design considerations spell the difference between an effective exhaust system and a weak one.

9. Are ducts clogged?
10. Does more than one hood exhaust into the same duct?
11. Is the fan enclosed?
12. Is the fan noisy?
13. Is makeup air supplied?
14. Is the makeup air treated (i.e., is it heated in the winter and cooled in the summer)?
15. Are drafts from other parts of the building (i.e., a nearby open window) interfering with the performance of the hood?
16. Is the system regularly cleaned and maintained?
17. Is the system running at full capacity?
18. Has the production process been changed without changing the ventilation system?

SOURCE: Food and Allied Service Trades Dept., AFL-CIO, 815 16th St., N.W., Washington, D.C. 20006. (202) 737-7200. Reprinted with permission.

One factor is how close the hood is located to the source of a contaminant. Even slight amounts of air turbulence, whether created by open windows or merely the movement of people, can push contaminants out of the range of the hood, which highlights the need for a shielded pathway into the exhaust system. Another important factor is how ducts are designed. Contaminants flow most effectively through short-run, large-diameter ducts and through ducts without elbow bends. Ducts should be corrosion resistant and free from holes and leaks.

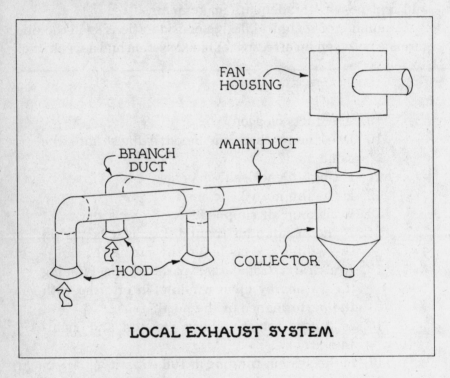

FAN HOUSING

BRANCH DUCT

MAIN DUCT

HOOD

COLLECTOR

LOCAL EXHAUST SYSTEM

What Goes Wrong

Poor design, installation, operation, or maintenance of HVAC and local ventilation systems, as well as contamination within the system itself, lie at the heart of most workplace pollution problems. Occasionally, faulty HVAC systems can cause disastrous problems. Twenty-two separate investigations have been launched at an infamous Washington, D.C., office building, where complaints about mold growth, auto exhaust contamination, water leaks, poor air distribution, and inadequate heating, cooling, and dehumidification have been heard for many years. While some investigators believe that bandage solutions—including better maintenance, decontamination of the coil units, and reduced humidity levels—can remedy the problem, others have concluded that without a complete overhaul of the HVAC system, the building will have to be abandoned.

The failure to adjust ventilation in response to changing circumstances is a common and less complex problem. For example, an HVAC system designed for a residential building is likely to be inappropriate if that building is converted to commercial uses. That's what happened at Columbia Plaza, a fourteen-story building near Washington's Kennedy Center, where mold growth became uncontrollable after apartment dwellers moved out and workers with the State Department and other government agencies moved in. Similarly, an exhaust vent that effectively removes fumes in a room with one printing press is probably inadequate for two. Introducing new office equipment, increasing the numbers of workers using the same space, or erecting new partitions or walls all call for adjustments to ensure that ventilation meets current needs.

Other problems trace back to the 1970s energy crisis and operational changes made to conserve and economize. In our earlier discussion of sick building syndrome, we described the rush to increase the use of recirculated air, at the expense of makeup air. Unless local exhaust is provided, odors and chemicals that initially posed problems only in a contained area can thus migrate unchecked, becoming the concern of entire floors and sometimes a whole building.

Reducing the entry of makeup air into the system, either in whole or in part, has other unintended consequences as well. If exhaust vents remain open while intake vents are blocked—allowing the amount of stale air being exhausted to exceed the intake of fresh air—a pressure imbalance is quickly created. Essentially a vacuum effect, negative pressure poses several hazards. Sometimes the flow of air reverses itself, and contaminated air is sucked back through the exhaust vents and recirculated into the ventilation system. Or a backdraft can be created in combustion flues, pulling carbon monoxide and other combustion by-products back into the passageways through which they were to have been expelled.

Another economy measure that has sometimes been employed is shutting down the HVAC system periodically, usually when the building is unoccupied. This sounds logical until we remember that outgassing, evaporation, and other contaminating processes take place even when no one is inside. If the air in a tightly sealed building has no outlet, contaminants accumulate and workers are certain to face problems with stuffy, polluted air as soon as they return to the office. In fact, what has traditionally been shrugged off as the Monday morning blues may actually be a physiological reaction to indoor air pollution. If the system is shut off periodically, it should not be until the building is emptied, and the system should be run for several hours before the building is reoccupied.

More than one air quality investigation has traced the source of pollution to malfunctioning intake vents. After absenteeism rates shot up at one Maryland firm, consultants were called in to determine why. They found high concentrations of dust, fiberglass, carbon monoxide, and fungus in the air and eventually discovered that the fresh air intake vents had not been opened for two years. Similar problems occur when vents are poorly positioned. In the corporate headquarters of one California firm, inspectors discovered that contaminated air being expelled through an exhaust vent was picked up by a nearby intake vent and circulated back through the building. Vents located near outdoor sources of pollution—downwind of an industrial smokestack, near loading docks, or close to a road with heavy traffic, for example—can also result in disastrous indoor pollution. Even when enough clean air is brought inside, not everyone in the workplace will be able to draw an equally fresh breath. The obstruction of airflow vents, often by employees whose desks are positioned too close to a strong current of hot or cold air, can sharply reduce air circulation. Improperly positioned file cabinets, office equipment, and room partitions can also create barriers to air movement that result in unbalanced ventilation.

Failing to schedule routine cleaning and maintenance of both HVAC and local ventilation systems allows contaminants, particularly bacteria and other microorganisms, to collect in ducts, air-cleaning filters, and dehumidifier drain pans. Clogged filters, improperly positioned hoods, and corroded ductwork can render local exhaust ventilation almost totally ineffective. Investigators have sometimes uncovered grizzly findings: A team of consultants at one firm discovered that rats had moved into the ductwork; birds' nests, snakes, cockroaches, and animal feces have also been reported.

All of these ventilation problems are intensified by the absence of state and local legislation. True, most municipalities have incorporated ventilation standards, such as those recommended by ASHRAE, into their building codes. And developers are expected to show blueprints and engineering plans in order to obtain permits and regulatory approval. But once ventilation system designs are approved, governmental oversight generally ends—and abuses sometimes begin. In Chapter 9 we'll look more closely at changes in public policy that could improve ventilation in commercial buildings.

CHEMICAL CONTAMINATION

A formidable concoction of chemicals in the workplace is generated from a variety of sources, including office processes, such as the use of machinery; human activities, such as cigarette smoking and ordinary respiration; and building materials and furnishings. Many of the contaminants found in office buildings will be familiar to students of residential pollution—carbon monoxide and formaldehyde are both in ample supply, as are volatile organic compounds (VOCs), which are generated primarily from the widespread use of solvents and pesticides. Other pollutants are unique to commercial buildings—ozone, for example, is associated primarily with photocopiers and other electrical equipment.

Here's a brief look at the polluters that contribute to chemical buildup in the workplace:

OFFICE FURNISHINGS AND BUILDING MATERIALS: A long list of materials used to construct and furnish office buildings can contaminate the air. Formaldehyde outgassing is the most common problem. Small wonder: The noxious gas is found in some 3,000 different building products. As in the home, sources of formaldehyde include furnishings, paneling and cabinetry made of particleboard and plywood, carpet, upholstered fabrics, drapery products, and urea-formaldehyde foam insulation. Outgassing is at its most intense during the first months of a product's life, although it can be detected at low levels indefinitely.

Other products associated with office renovations, including paints, varnishes, shellacs, and the solvents used to thin or clean them, as well as the adhesives in recently installed carpeting, emit a range of VOCs. The problem is particularly acute during and immediately after construction, before fumes fully dissipate.

Because the dangers of radon exposure are most acute in the office building's basement and on the ground floor, where relatively few workers are likely to spend substantial amounts of time, concern over the radioactive gas is not as great in the workplace as in the home. Occasionally, however, radon emitted from construction materials such as concrete, brick, and stone may accumulate to levels sufficient to be a health risk.

Other potential sources of contamination include the plastic panels used to create room dividers, which release dimethyl acetamide, known to cause tearing of the eyes; fiber particles from building insulation, which are a skin irritant; duct and pipe insulation and acoustical tiles, which release polyvinyl chloride; and electrical transformers, which emit PCBs.

PHOTOCOPIERS AND OTHER OFFICE MACHINES: Photocopying machines and other common electrical equipment give off ozone, a pungent gas that can cause eye, nose, and throat irritation even at low doses. At higher doses, exposure results in coughing, chest pains, and fatigue; chronic exposure to ozone can eventually cause lung disease. Well-maintained and properly ventilated photocopiers rarely exceed OSHA's safety threshold of 0.1 ppm and are unlikely to produce any of these health effects, but a strong odor in the room suggests that OSHA limits are being exceeded. An immediate inspection should be sought. The toners and other chemicals used in the photocopying process also present hazards to the worker in the form of respirable vapors and dust particles. Additionally, sensitive individuals may develop a rash from handling chemical-laden photocopy paper.

Other polluting office equipment includes blueprint machines, which release ammonia; photographic equipment, which releases acetic acid; and spirit duplicators, which release methyl alcohol.

OFFICE SUPPLIES: A host of quotidian office supplies—including felt-tip marker pens, glue, and rubber cement—contain toxic VOCs such as benzene, toluene, styrene, trichlorethylene, and carbon tetrachloride. In California, one manufacturer of typewriter correction fluid is being pressured either to change the product's chemical formulation or to warn consumers that it contains a known carcinogen.

Other toxins are contained in carbonless carbon paper, which gives off PCBs, and in conventional carbon paper, typewriter ribbons, and inks, which all contain solvents that can irritate the skin and produce chemical-rich fumes.

CLEANING AGENTS: Cleaning products and solvents are as ubiquitous in the workplace as they are in the home. Unless the ventilation system is performing at its peak and great care is taken to use the products according to manufacturer's instructions, many volatile organic compounds linger in the air after evaporating from disinfectants, ammonia-based cleansers, carpet shampoos, and floor waxes. Industrial-strength cleaners are particularly likely to leave an irritating residue in the carpets, especially if they are inadequately diluted.

COMBUSTION BY-PRODUCTS: Unwelcome by-products of the combustion process, including carbon monoxide and sulfur dioxide, can invade from outside the building, especially if HVAC intake vents are located near a loading dock or another source of automobile emissions. The contaminating by-products of heating fuels and gas stoves (which are less common than in the home but still present in some workplaces) generally originate inside the building.

As we've already explored in detail, cigarette smoke is one of the leading contaminants of indoor air, exposing both smokers and nonsmokers to a lengthy list of carcinogens and other toxic chemicals.

PESTICIDES: Thousands of pesticides, formed from a combination of 1,800 different active ingredients, are commercially available, although 90 percent of them are used for agricultural purposes. In the workplace, pesticides are commonly sprayed on plants and throughout the premises to rid them of mites, cockroaches, and other undesirable insects. Typically, the concentrations used are more toxic than in the home. The residue of hazardous chemicals left by these pesticides can be absorbed through the skin, ingested, or inhaled, eventually accumulating in the fatty tissues of the body.

Health-associated problems depend on the particular chemical components, but a number of common pesticide ingredients are suspected carcinogens or have been shown to be highly toxic in laboratory tests. Three of the most prevalent indoor pesticides are chlordane, sulfuryl fluoride, and chlorpyrifos. Chlordane, the most commonly used pesticide in the country until the 1970s, has finally been banned from all use by the Environmental Protection Agency. Until 1987, however, it was still being used as a termiticide, and traces of the toxic chemical linger. Sulfuryl fluoride is used as a fumigant, a class of pesticides that have "extraordinary power to penetrate the lining membrane of the respiratory and gastrointestinal tracts, and the skin," according to the EPA. Chlorpyrifos, labeled "moderately toxic" by the agency, is often associated with sick building syndrome.

BIOLOGICAL CONTAMINATION

Staff members at the Department of Health and Human Services, located in the Hubert H. Humphrey Building in Washington, D.C., can be counted among the victims of biological contamination spread by the HVAC system. In the mid-1980s, outbreaks of flulike symptoms periodically swept through the office, seemingly without cause, until a water leak was discovered in pipes hidden behind the office walls. It was not long before investigators realized that moisture had soaked into the office carpeting and furniture, allowing bacteria and fungi to reproduce unchecked, enter the ventilation system, and cause widespread affliction.

That's not an uncommon story. The ability of mold and other biological contaminants to flourish in the presence of excess condensation, high humidity, and stagnant water has already been described. In addition to leaks, flush toilets, humidifiers, ice machines, and even old books, damp newsprint, and rarely used files are popular gathering spots for microorganisms.

Various components of the HVAC system also allow for biological growth unless they are properly maintained. Filters used to clean both recirculated and fresh outdoor air readily become breeding grounds unless they are changed regularly. In the humidification process, water drains into sumps, where it must be treated or replaced with fresh water to avoid contamination. Similarly, dehumidifier drain pans beneath the cooling coils are a ready source of stagnant water unless they are emptied regularly.

Once microorganisms begin to grow, they can enter the ventilation system and spread into every room in the building. Legionnaire's disease, of course, is the most infamous consequence of microbial contamination, but hypersensitivity pneumonitis and humidifier fever are much more common. Typically, the symptoms disappear when workers leave the building and recur soon after they return. Tracing these problems to their roots is not always easy because any number of bacteria, fungi, protozoa, or other microbes can cause illness; in at least one large office building, containment efforts generated several million dollars in repair bills.

A WORD ABOUT ASBESTOS

The insulating and fire retarding capacities of asbestos make the product as widely used in the workplace as it is in the home. In commercial buildings, asbestos can be found in acoustic ceiling and floor tiles; pipe, duct, and boiler insulation; and ventilation shafts. The so-called miracle fiber is also contained in countless plastics, textiles, insulating and decorative products, and construction materials.

Friable asbestos, the crumbly variety that is most likely to emit fibers into the air, is present in some 20 percent of office buildings, according to a ten-city Environmental Protection Agency study. Just how great is the accompanying danger? The EPA took a count and concluded that occupa-

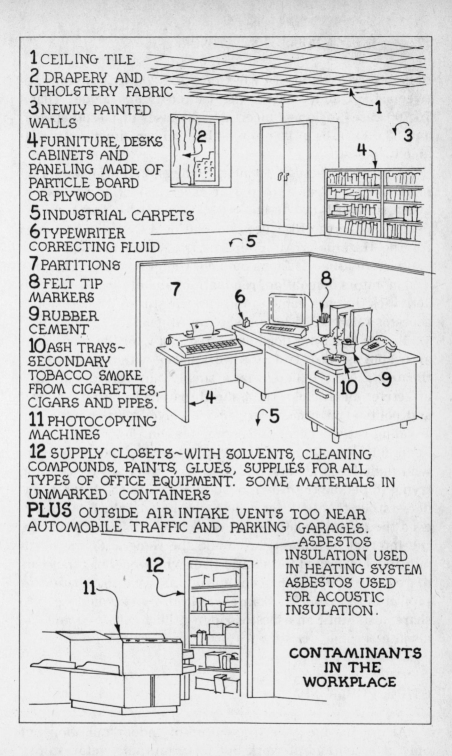

1 CEILING TILE

2 DRAPERY AND UPHOLSTERY FABRIC

3 NEWLY PAINTED WALLS

4 FURNITURE, DESKS CABINETS AND PANELING MADE OF PARTICLE BOARD OR PLYWOOD

5 INDUSTRIAL CARPETS

6 TYPEWRITER CORRECTING FLUID

7 PARTITIONS

8 FELT TIP MARKERS

9 RUBBER CEMENT

10 ASH TRAYS~ SECONDARY TOBACCO SMOKE FROM CIGARETTES, CIGARS AND PIPES.

11 PHOTOCOPYING MACHINES

12 SUPPLY CLOSETS~WITH SOLVENTS, CLEANING COMPOUNDS, PAINTS, GLUES, SUPPLIES FOR ALL TYPES OF OFFICE EQUIPMENT. SOME MATERIALS IN UNMARKED CONTAINERS

PLUS OUTSIDE AIR INTAKE VENTS TOO NEAR AUTOMOBILE TRAFFIC AND PARKING GARAGES.

ASBESTOS INSULATION USED IN HEATING SYSTEM ASBESTOS USED FOR ACOUSTIC INSULATION.

CONTAMINANTS IN THE WORKPLACE

tional asbestos exposure will cause 131,200 extra deaths between 1985 and 2009 in the United States alone. That's
76,700 cases of lung cancer, 21,500 cases of mesothelioma,
and 33,000 cases of gastrointestinal cancer directly attribut-
able to asbestos.

Because of these and similar findings, various federal regulations have been targeted at asbestos in the workplace.
OSHA standards are designed to limit on-the-job asbestos exposure, while the EPA uses the National Emission Standard
for the Hazardous Air Pollutant (NESHAP) to control the
emission of asbestos fibers outside. Under NESHAP, the EPA
also monitors demolition, renovation, and other construction
activities that are liable to disturb asbestos. (For more about
asbestos-related legislation, see the Appendix.)

But no federal official has dared lobby for the removal of
all friable asbestos from the workplace—with a price tag estimated at $51 billion, that's simply not considered cost-
effective. Meanwhile, the issue threatens to become a legal
and political nightmare, with all involved parties intent on
avoiding responsibility for contamination. For example, the
Federal Reserve Bank of Minneapolis is suing the contractors
who built its landmark building. And they are considering
trying to peddle their own headquarters—to the highest bid-
der—rather than pay for asbestos removal, which might exceed the original construction costs of $34 million. Similarly,
the Internal Revenue Service and the General Services Administration argued for months over who would pay the costs
of relocating IRS employees during an asbestos abatement
project in Pine Bluff, Arkansas. Neither party would agree to
share costs until an asbestos-laden ceiling collapsed and the
dispute became a crisis.

OTHER PUBLIC SPACES

Americans face the discomfort of indoor pollution not
only at home and at work but in restaurants, retail stores,

public transportation, and any other public space where contaminants are released into the air and ventilation is inadequate. The problem is particularly acute where smokers mingle with nonsmokers—many states and municipalities still do not mandate separate smoking sections in restaurants or bars, for example. On airplanes, where lowering ventilation rates reduces fuel use, passengers frequently complain about the poor quality of the air. And in America's ubiquitous indoor shopping malls, tightly sealed buildings, the absence of windows, and improperly designed HVAC systems create problems analogous to those in the workplace.

Fortunately, we don't spend many concentrated hours in any of these places, and short-term exposure is unlikely to do much harm. However, there is greater cause for alarm in two other public spaces: schools and hospitals.

Schools

Because their bodies are still developing and their respiration rates are faster than those of adults, children are thought to be particularly vulnerable to pollution-related health hazards. Two stories illustrate why so many parents are concerned about the safety of the school environment.

In the midst of a $20 million renovation project at the elite Boston Latin School, a number of students and teachers became violently ill and had to be sent home. Construction was brought to a halt, and city inspectors found that the air had been poisoned by fumes from solvents and other chemical agents. Contractors were required to hire an engineering consultant and to improve safety procedures before proceeding with the renovations.

Another incident took place in an Arizona elementary school, which was evacuated after occupants complained of irritation, headaches, and stomach pain. Some $200,000 was allocated to test the air, install environmental monitoring equipment, and improve drainage. To be certain the building was safe, adult volunteers were then asked to spend two eight-hour periods sitting in the classrooms before the school was reopened to children.

Considerable attention has also been paid to the importance of protecting children from asbestos. In response to intense political pressure, the federal government passed the Asbestos Hazard Emergency Response Act in 1986, which requires all local school districts to inspect their facilities for both friable and nonfriable asbestos-containing materials. If asbestos is found, the school board is then required to develop an action plan for its control or removal. The cost of identifying and replacing asbestos products in schools is hefty—the price tag for asbestos removal in the Chicago area alone has been estimated at $1 billion.

Lead poisoning, which can stunt development or cause retardation, is another grave risk for young children. Most exposure comes from lead-based paints or airborne lead expelled from automobile exhaust, but in the schools attention is particularly focused on lead-lined water coolers. Under the Lead Contamination Control Act of 1988 such coolers have been banned, although they remain in widespread use. Other provisions of the legislation expand a lead screening program for children and direct the EPA to assist schools in testing their facilities for lead.

Radon is an additional and sobering threat in the schools, and the EPA has called for testing in all educational facilities. Other pollution hazards are associated with special classroom activities, such as chemistry and biology labs and art classes, where toxic contaminants can build unless appropriate ventilation is provided. Tight budgets can also contribute indirectly to pollution problems—when a choice must be made between slashing programs and reducing ventilation system maintenance, school boards tend to opt for maintenance cuts that are perceived as noncontroversial.

Hospitals

Sadly, there is wisdom in the old saw that hospitals are no place for the sick. The contaminating processes that take place in hospitals surpass those found in ordinary commercial buildings: Along with the usual suspects emitted from building materials and furnishings, cigarette smoking, and cleaning agents, hospitals generate chemical pollutants from laboratory and surgical procedures, combustion by-products from institutional cooking, and aerosol particles from the large volume of laundry done on the premises. VOC-rich air fresheners, disinfectants, and anesthetic gases are also likely to be used in unusually large quantities.

Yet HVAC systems are no more likely to be properly maintained in hospitals than they are in office buildings. While sterilization procedures usually prevent epidemics from racing through hospital corridors, the occasional spread of contagious diseases is well documented. In one Florida clinic, health workers were exposed to tuberculosis in part because building ventilation was inadequate. Poor filtration and the minimal entry of makeup air (more than 90 percent of the air in the HVAC system was recirculated) allowed the tuberculin bacteria to spread outward from a room in which infected AIDS patients were being treated.

Whether the public space is an office, a hospital, a school, or even the waiting room of an airport, indoor pollution can create problems in any environment where people gather, especially when only minimal fresh air is available. The good news, though, is that there are ways to clean up most indoor spaces and breathe free again.

8
A NEW WAY TO WORK
Steps Toward
a Healthier Office

Employees are generally the first to be affected by work site pollution and the most vociferous in pressuring for change. "The burden of proof is generally put on the employee," says health and safety expert Jim Duffy, who has investigated scores of complaints from AT&T workers in New York City on behalf of their union, the Communications Workers of America (CWA). In a sad commentary on today's business climate, Duffy attributes the dearth of employer initiatives in this area to the fact that "doing something about asbestos doesn't show up in the balance sheet for the next quarter."

At EPA headquarters, where some 100 employees have fallen victim to sick building syndrome, much the same complaint has been made: "I believe that if management had initially taken the problem seriously and taken immediate action under the terms of its own indoor air policy, we could have been spared the trauma and distress of this illness," said Steve Shapiro, an EPA employee.

Despite resistance, however, employer cooperation in the sometimes-complex task of solving indoor air quality problems is crucial. Employee determination, good organizing skills, and strong leadership are all necessary to remind employers of their stake in eliminating building pollution. One forceful argument is that productivity drops markedly when air quality is poor. Absenteeism and even turnover rates, which both have a direct impact on the employer's pocketbook, also rise in sick buildings. And the skyrocketing costs of medical care, a major corporate expense, are inevitably affected by the air quality in the workplace.

ASSESSING THE PROBLEM

Whether the work is done by an employee committee, the building maintenance staff, or professional consultants, here's what investigators will need to do when indoor air quality problems are reported:

- Document employee health complaints.
- Examine architectural blueprints, floor plans, and ventilation system specifications.
- Walk through the work site, looking at the building's layout, the position of room dividers, and the location of vent ducts.
- Test for contaminants.
- Develop a plan for reducing or eliminating pollution problems.

As an employee, you have the right to be kept informed throughout the investigation as well as when final recommendations are made. You should also be supplied with background material about indoor pollution, available from a number of government agencies and unions, to help you become aware of your risks, to encourage you to take common-sense precautions, and to provide you with a greater sense of control over your environment.

Bring in an Expert

The often-adversarial relationship between employees and employers sometimes interferes with a teamwork approach to solving air quality problems. Rather than risk an escalating conflict, companies often seek help from objective outsiders.

Fortunately, there are lots of experts available. Sick building syndrome and related problems have spawned teams of specialists known as indoor air quality consultants who are drawn from the ranks of engineers, environmental hygienists, chemists, and microbiologists. Private consultants are costly, however. Analyzing indoor air quality problems and testing a building's HVAC system can run upwards of $3,000, for example—and that doesn't include specialized testing or the costs of cleanup.

A less expensive alternative is to request a free investigation from the National Institute for Occupational Safety and Health (NIOSH), a federal agency associated with the Centers for Disease Control. Since 1971, NIOSH has entered more than 500 work sites, usually at the invitation of employee groups, unions, management, and other government agencies, to make recommendations for improving indoor air quality. Specific federal regulations describe how NIOSH must assess evaluation requests, mandate employer cooperation, and establish action procedures when imminent danger is detected. One of its biggest projects to date, undertaken in conjunction with other public and private agencies, is determining what has gone wrong with the James Madison Memorial Building, a part of the Library of Congress, in Washington, D.C. Employees have been grumbling about air quality for ten years and an in-depth, two-year study should tell us why.

Unfortunately, NIOSH's limited resources do not allow investigators to visit the site of every problem. Call the toll-free number, listed in the Appendix, to find out if your building site qualifies and to get other valuable guidance.

Document Employee Health Complaints

Once investigators have been selected, the formal evaluation process begins with a systematic survey of all workers. Questionnaires asking employees about the nature, severity, and chronology of their symptoms and discomfort are generally distributed. Personal interviews may also be conducted to flesh out the responses and to secure anecdotal information. "It's just like journalism," says CWA expert Jim Duffy. "You have to get the who, what, why, where, when, and how of the situation."

The objective of the information-gathering process is to

determine when health problems occur, to find out who is most susceptible and why, to pinpoint the building areas in which problems are most acute, and to establish a definitive link between illness and office air quality. At one twenty-five-story state office building in Virginia, a startling 55 percent of questionnaire respondents said they had symptoms of discomfort that worsened while in the building; most of these individuals had missed some work as a result.

An analysis of employee responses helps provide a clearer picture of the cause of the problem. A particularly useful activity is to plot the location of employees who express the most severe complaints on an office floor plan. This helps to determine whether the problem is widespread or localized and whether it can clearly be associated with particular office equipment in the vicinity.

A sample questionnaire, to be completed by all employees in problem areas, is included here.

Employee Questionnaire

Here are the questions that workers need to be asked when a building is being evaluated for indoor air quality problems:

1. What health complaints have you experienced at work?
2. Do you have any of the following conditions?
   Hay fever ____
   Other allergies ____
   Dermatitis or other skin problems ____
   Sinus problems ____
   Colds or flu ____
   Nausea or dizziness ____
   Eye irritation ____
   Headache ____
   Excess fatigue ____
   Joint aches ____

3. When did you first notice these symptoms?

4. When do the symptoms occur? How often?

5. Do your symptoms clear up within an hour of leaving work? If not, which symptoms persist through the week?

6. Are the symptoms more likely to appear at particular times of the day?

7. Do they occur in particular areas of the building?

8. How many co-workers smoke? Do you smoke?

9. Is there a specific incident to which your health problems can be traced (i.e., building renovations, installation of new carpeting, purchase of new furniture)?

10. What office machines are used in your vicinity? What chemicals do they use?

11. What office products are used that contain chemicals? List the ingredients.

12. What fabrics are used in the carpets, curtains, shades, and wall coverings? Is there any evidence of excessive dust or mold?

13. Are you aware of any water leaks in the building that have not been repaired promptly?

14. What is your overall assessment of the air quality and comfort level in your office?

15. Do you work with any office equipment? Specify the type.

16. Where is your office located? Specify floor, department, and proximity to office equipment.

17. How old are you?

18. What is your job title? Briefly describe your responsibilities.

19. What is the general condition of your health?

20. Is there any family history of illness?

Study the Building

Collecting data on the character of the building and its air-handling systems is an important means of identifying the source of indoor pollution problems. The cooperation of an engineer or building maintenance staff will be extremely helpful. Often, the staff will be asked to complete a different questionnaire, one focusing on the building itself. A sample questionnaire is included below.

Before a walk-through inspection begins, it is best to determine the following:

- Who is responsible for the operation and maintenance of the HVAC system?
- Where are the manufacturer's design specifications? If design specs or standard operating procedures are in writing, copies should be supplied to the investigators.
- What procedures are followed if the ventilation system fails to operate properly?

A great deal can be learned about indoor air quality simply by walking through the office and making careful observations. Not all pollutants emit an odor, but a strong smell certainly suggests a problem. Sometimes an irritant is severe enough to bring tears to the eyes of anyone who walks into the room. Dust particles that settle on work surfaces, the presence of stagnant water, office equipment without adequate ventilation, and air temperature that is obviously too cold or too hot all hint at possible pollution problems. At the Virginia office building, investigators noticed microbial growth near the HVAC system and in personal humidifiers, improperly stored gasoline cans, and construction in process on several floors.

The HVAC system also should be inspected to determine whether intake and exhaust vents are provided in every room and whether air flows continuously through these vents. Holding a tissue at the face of each vent is an easy way to test air movement. The position of the supply and exhaust vents relative to each other is an important consideration—

when they are too close together, clean, fresh air may be pulled out the exhaust vent as soon as it enters the room. If the room has been partitioned, it will be important to walk through each one of the cubicles to determine whether the barriers prevent vented air from circulating properly. The duct-work and other contaminant-prone components of the HVAC system also should be inspected.

Finally, local ventilation systems should be scrutinized to determine their effectiveness. The questionnaire provided in the previous chapter is a useful reference for evaluating a local exhaust system.

About the Building

The National Institute for Occupational Safety and Health has developed the following questionnaire for use by concerned employee groups, employers, or its own investigators:

1. How old is the building?
2. What construction materials have been used?
3. How many floors in the building? How many square feet per floor?
4. What types of windows are in the building? Do they open?
5. Who is responsible for the functioning of the building systems?
6. Who is responsible for cleaning the interior of the building? How often is the building cleaned?
7. Have there been any major renovations or operating changes? What were they? When did they occur?
8. Does the building have sprayed or foamed insulation? When was it applied?

9. What type of heating system is used?

10. What type of cooling system is used?

11. What type of humidification system is used?

12. How is the total ventilation system operated?

13. What floors and rooms are served by each system?

14. What type of filtration system is used? How often is it changed or maintenanced?

15. How much fresh air is being introduced into the ventilation system? Does this amount meet system specifications?

16. Where are the fresh air inlets? Are they functioning properly?

17. Are there any possible sources of contamination located in the general vicinity of the air inlets?

18. How likely are contaminants to be drawn into the air inlets due to prevailing winds and inversions?

19. How does exhaust air leave the building?

20. Is the building being used for the same purpose for which it was designed?

21. What types of activities are building occupants engaged in?

22. What processes or activities are present in the building that may serve as contaminant sources? Is local exhaust ventilation used near contamination sources?

SOURCE: Hazard Evaluations and Technical Assistance Branch, National Institute for Occupational Safety and Health, 4676 Columbia Pkwy., Cincinnati, Ohio 45226. (513) 841-4374. Reprinted with permission.

Testing for Contaminants

Finally, environmental monitoring begins. Some basic screening tests can help provide fast feedback to concerned employees. Easy-to-use instruments include a detector tube for measuring carbon dioxide levels, a velometer for measuring the strength of airflow, and a smoke tube for determining air movement. Measuring room temperature and humidity at various times and places throughout the day helps determine room comfort and the overall efficiency of the HVAC system.

More complex tests for specific chemical and microbial contaminants can also be run. Sometimes the findings of such tests create more problems than they solve, however. Concentration levels of specific contaminants typically turn out to be well below the maximum standards established for the workplace (which are often more applicable to factories than to office buildings), yet findings of "acceptable" levels tempt building owners to dismiss air quality complaints. Before such tests are run, therefore, it is important to remind all participants that building-related illnesses are commonly caused by low-level accumulation of many toxic substances, not high levels of a single contaminant. No single contaminant was found to be at unusually high levels in the Virginia office building.

CARBON DIOXIDE DETECTOR TUBES: Monitoring the level of carbon dioxide, which is exhaled, is a useful gauge of ventilation efficiency. While carbon dioxide alone does not result in discomfort or health complaints, its presence at high concentrations suggests that other, more virulent contaminants are also likely to be present. Ambient outdoor levels of carbon dioxide are usually about 250 to 300 parts per million (ppm). That figure soars indoors—if concentration levels are kept at about 600 ppm or below, complaints about air quality are usually minimal. Above 1,000 ppm, however, typical sick building symptoms, such as headache, fatigue, and eye, nose, and throat irritation, may be present.

Carbon dioxide detector tubes, which can be purchased

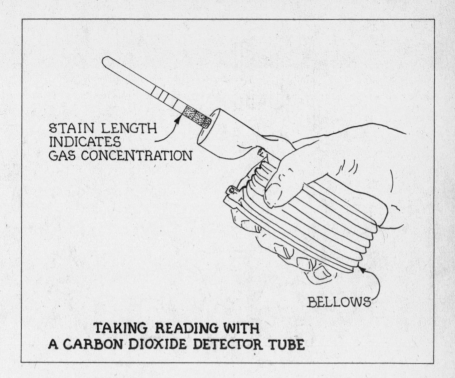

STAIN LENGTH
INDICATES
GAS CONCENTRATION

BELLOWS

TAKING READING WITH
A CARBON DIOXIDE DETECTOR TUBE

at industrial safety equipment supply houses, indicate gas concentration by the length of a colored stain on a metered tube. Readings should be taken at several locations, both where problems have been reported and where they have not. Baseline sampling should begin early in the morning, when the building is mostly unoccupied, at all major test spots. Further readings should be taken at each location several times during the day, and all measurements should be recorded by location, time of day, and nature of the activities taking place.

SMOKE TUBES: A smoke tube, sold in any hardware store, is an easy and effective way to monitor the direction of airflow or to identify "dead spaces" where still air allows pollutants to accumulate. A smoke tube is a small, plastic tube with a rubber squeeze ball at one end. The tube is filled with a harmless, lightweight chemical powder and when the bulb

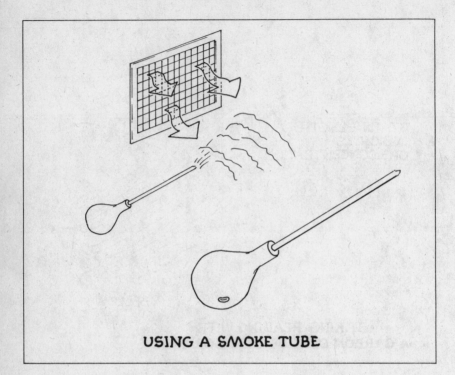

USING A SMOKE TUBE

is squeezed, chemical smoke floats into the air. The movement of the smoke shows whether a room exhaust vent or the hood of a local exhaust system is working properly. Drafts and air turbulence can be observed by watching the smoke.

VELOMETERS: An inexpensive gadget also known as an airflow meter, a velometer measures the flow of air past a particular point in feet per minute. One device is commonly attached to a supply vent to measure air intake, while another is secured to an exhaust vent or hood near the source of a contaminant to determine how quickly contaminants are being exhausted.

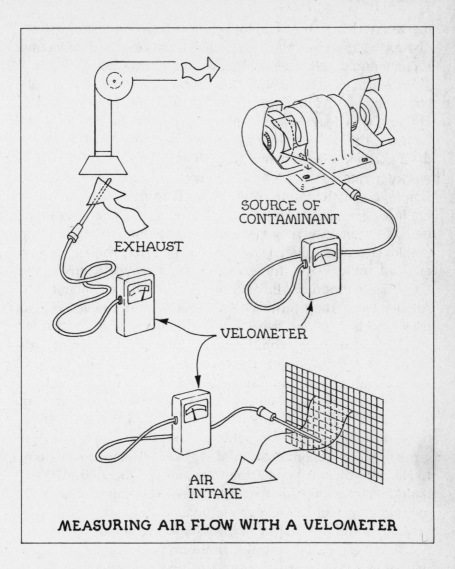

MEASURING AIR FLOW WITH A VELOMETER

IMPLEMENTING SOLUTIONS

Once a thorough assessment of office air quality problems has been made, concrete steps must be taken to solve them. Otherwise, employee resentment is inevitable: There's nothing worse than asking employees to complete questionnaires, disrupting the workplace with investigations, and collecting recommendations—then failing to follow through.

Sometimes investigations turn up easy solutions to clear-cut problems. At one work site, it was obvious that the machinery was leaking ammonia and had to be repaired; in another, the conclusion was quickly reached that a separate drying room was needed to prevent graphic artists from working right on top of their recently spray-painted signs. Employee participation often pays off at this stage. If workers have been kept informed about indoor air pollution problems, they may have some sound suggestions to offer. Once employees in an advertising firm learned that rubber cement emitted toxic VOCs, for example, they stopped purchasing large-size containers. Instead of pouring rubber cement into smaller cans, they purchased the small cans themselves, in bulk quantity, which was just as economical and a lot safer.

Often, however, solutions are trickier to pinpoint: Although fumes in one office were potent enough to make it virtually uninhabitable, industrial hygienists were unable to detect unusually high levels of a single pollutant. In that case, an analysis of the ventilation system revealed that more fresh outdoor air had to be brought into the building. In the Virginia building, a combination of steps was deemed necessary to clean up the air. In addition to recommending better HVAC maintenance, compliance with ASHRAE ventilation standards, and more careful housekeeping, investigators advised follow-up studies and the sharing of information with employees.

As in residential settings, there are four important steps necessary for correcting or preventing most indoor pollution problems:

1. Provide adequate ventilation.
2. Eliminate or control biological contamination.
3. Eliminate or control chemical contamination.
4. Restrict or ban smoking.

Solving Common Ventilation Problems

Minor alterations in HVAC design, tighter maintenance standards, and revised operational specifications are commonly all that is needed to bring air quality up to snuff. For instance, Itel Corporation spent just $5,000 to improve the ventilation system of an energy-efficient building in Port Washington, New York, where a combination of cigarette smoke, formaldehyde, and photocopier fumes had forced the evacuation of 150 employees.

A firm commitment to make necessary changes must be secured from the building owner, and assistance from maintenance personnel and other technicians is also imperative. A program of preventive maintenance and regular inspections should be established for all ventilation equipment. At a minimum, the rate at which fresh air enters the building and flows through occupied spaces should be measured regularly. Vents should be checked to be sure they are open, and filters should be replaced at regular intervals to prevent clogs that block airflow. Ductwork, drains below cooling coils, cooling tower water, and other components of the HVAC's humidification and dehumidification systems should be cleaned to prevent the growth of bacteria and fungi. Without this precaution, HVAC systems do more than fail to purge the air of contaminants: They actually contribute to the problems of polluted air.

Here are some solutions to other common ventilation system problems:

PROBLEM: The amount of fresh outdoor air that enters the ventilation system is inadequate. As a result, a vacuum effect allows the airflow to reverse itself through the exhaust vents and stale air circulates through the building.

SOLUTION: Check that the louvers that allow fresh air to enter from outdoors are open and functioning properly. If no blockage is evident, the HVAC system may need to be adjusted to increase the ratio of fresh to recirculated air. Professional engineering help is usually needed to correct this imbalance.

PROBLEM: Intake vents are pulling contaminated air into the building.

SOLUTION: An extensive revamping of the ventilation system is often required to solve this problem, which usually results from improperly positioned intake and exhaust vents. Intake vents located downwind of exhaust vents, for example, can capture air being expelled and send it back into the building; automobile fumes or industrial wastes can also be pulled inside. Expert advice may be needed to reconfigure the system so that only clean makeup air is allowed to enter.

PROBLEM: Some HVAC systems are designed to reduce the intake of fresh air when indoor temperatures reach a certain level; lowered airflow results in inefficient contaminant removal.

SOLUTION: Airflow specifications should be determined not only by the temperature desired at the workplace but by ventilation requirements. The system may need to be modified so that sufficient fresh air continues to enter the building even when temperatures are optimal.

PROBLEM: Fresh air is not circulating properly through all parts of an indoor space.

SOLUTION: All air vents inside the building should be checked regularly to ensure that they are open and unobstructed. Employees should not be asked to sit near a direct stream of air, which may be uncomfortably hot or cold, and they should be educated to the consequences of blocking air supply registers in an effort to control room temperature. If room dividers, partitions, or new walls are erected, maintenance staff should check to see that adequate airflow still reaches all parts of the office.

PROBLEM: A ventilation system may operate only when a building is fully occupied or be shut down before most workers leave for the night, allowing building-generated pollutants, such as formaldehyde, to accumulate for many hours.

SOLUTION: The ventilation system should be set to run for several hours before workers enter the building for the day and should not be turned off until the building has been emptied. If maintenance personnel or other employees often burn the midnight oil at the office, the system may need to operate around the clock.

Controlling Chemical Contamination

Unfortunately, it's not practical to eliminate many of the synthetics which are so crucial to the efficient functioning of the modern office. A more realistic objective is to learn about the hazards of common workplace materials, to make substitutions when possible, and to assure that local and general ventilation systems, the most effective means of controlling chemical contamination, are working at their full potential.

Many of the specific solutions recommended earlier for ridding residences of volatile organic compounds, including formaldehyde, are equally relevant in the workplace. Here are some additional pointers:

- Photocopying equipment should be well ventilated and set apart from densely populated office areas so that workers do not breathe excessive chemical fumes. A pungent odor is a sign that ozone levels are exceeding OSHA safety standards and should prompt a careful inspection. A regular schedule for cleaning and maintenance should be followed.
- Sensitive individuals prone to skin rashes should wear protective gloves when handling photocopier paper or using cleaners and other solvents.
- Smokers should be segregated from nonsmokers and ventilation rates may need to be increased. See "Restricting Smoking at the Workplace," page 193 for more details on corporate smoking policies.

- When possible, the use of toxic solvents rich in hazardous VOCs should be avoided. Employees should get into the habit of reading labels and advocate for the purchase of nontoxic substitutes. If there is no good substitute, cleaning should be scheduled when few workers are present, and the office should be thoroughly ventilated during and after cleaning.
- Lobby to have building ventilation rates increased for the first months after formaldehyde-rich products are installed, when outgassing rates are highest. Unfortunately, workers are unlikely to be given a choice between costly solid-wood products and inexpensive pressed wood, although the former is obviously less contaminating.
- Pesticides should be applied only when the building is unoccupied. Again, thorough ventilation is critical.

When new equipment is introduced or an office is renovated, pollutants are likely to rise to unusually high levels and special short-term measures should be implemented. Painting, the installation of new carpeting, and other construction is best scheduled in the evenings, on weekends, or whenever the building is least likely to be occupied. Physical barriers, such as temporary partitions or even a blockade of file cabinets, should be erected around construction areas to seal them off as much as possible. Ideally, adjustments can be made to enhance local ventilation while keeping pollutants from circulating through the rest of the building.

The highest concentration of contaminants should be dispersed before workers are moved into a newly renovated area. Running an exhaust system around the clock in the first weeks during and after the completion of construction activities will greatly speed pollutant dispersal. Baking off contaminants by temporarily raising room temperature is a technique that shows some promise, but researchers say its effectiveness remains unproven.

Reducing Biological Contamination

As in the home, maintaining low relative humidity levels and establishing good cleanliness and maintenance habits will go a long way toward eliminating microbial breeding grounds and discouraging biological growth. In addition, pools of standing water should not be allowed to collect for long periods of time. A collaborative effort should be made by staff and supervisors to detect and repair water leaks—everyone should know where to report leaks, and maintenance personnel should be prepared to take prompt corrective action. If significant water damage does occur in an office building, porous carpets, furnishings, and ceiling tiles may have to be discarded. A simple cleaning is rarely efficient to eliminate microbial contamination here.

Nonporous surfaces where microbial growth is evident, such as HVAC system drain pans and cooling coils, should be cleaned and disinfected with detergents or bleach. These cleansers, which themselves can contaminate the air, should be thoroughly rinsed off before the HVAC system is turned back on. Drain pans under air-handling units also should be emptied regularly.

RESTRICTING SMOKING AT THE WORKPLACE

Smoking at the workplace has been well established as a major source of indoor pollution, and pressure to implement restrictions often originates with employees unable to work comfortably in a smoke-filled office environment. There is plenty of legal precedent for imposing anti-smoking rules, and a range of policies, running the gamut from highly restrictive to relatively permissive, can be tailored to any workplace.

Here's a closer look at what the law says about smoking and how workplace policies can be implemented.

Legal Precedents

An analysis of court decisions dealing with smoking, undertaken by the American Lung Association and detailed in *A Decision Maker's Guide to Reducing Smoking at the Worksite*, indicates that employers who fail to develop adequate smoking policies may actually be held liable for subsequent employee health problems. Among the findings:

- Employers can be held responsible for smoking-related illnesses of employees permitted to smoke on the job. In one California case (*Fuentes* v. *Workmen's Compensation Appeals Board*) an employer had to pay one-third the costs of an employee's disability because that employee was permitted to smoke on the job and thus "to inflict harm on himself."
- An employer's obligation to provide a safe workplace includes protecting the rights of nonsmokers, according to a 1976 New Jersey Supreme Court decision (*Shrimp* v. *New Jersey Bell*). The court held that "the right of an individual to risk his or her health does not include the right to jeopardize the health of those who must remain around him or her in order to properly perform the duties of their job." In a similar case in Washington, D.C., in 1988, the court ruled that an employer had failed to provide a safe workplace and had caused emotional distress to a nonsmoker.
- In the absence of a union contract mandating the right to smoke, the courts have consistently confirmed the rights of employers to restrict or ban smoking at the workplace. There are no legal grounds for the claim that smoking at work is an absolute "right."
- Employers have the right to refuse to hire smokers, as long as the policy is applied equitably.

Implementing a Smoking Policy

Regardless of legal precedents, however, creating a fair and viable smoking policy at the workplace is a tricky task.

In order to implement a policy that does not create undue dissension or resentment within the ranks, restrictions must be spelled out clearly and in writing. Employees need to know exactly where they can and cannot smoke and how the policies will be enforced. The company's rationale for imposing new rules should be explained in a memo or at a meeting, and exceptions must not be granted—a policy cannot work unless management, staff, and visitors are all subjected to the same rules. The company should also offer employees the opportunity to participate in stop-smoking sessions.

Smoking policies can be grouped into many categories, depending on their objectives:

- Policies designed to protect equipment or property. Many policies were initially developed to protect company property, but as the dangers of passive smoking became clear, they were viewed as favoring things more than people and were looked upon with disfavor.
- Policies designed to comply with laws or regulations. A growing number of states and municipalities insist that smoking be regulated in public places, forcing many firms to develop rules in compliance with local laws.
- Policies banning smoking in specific areas. Probably the most common policy used today, smoking bans generally are in effect in such areas as cafeterias, bathrooms, conference rooms, and auditoriums. These are important, but rather minimal, restrictions; nonsmokers are still forced to breathe air fouled by cigarettes through most of the workplace.
- Policies confining smoking to specific areas. Unless otherwise designated, the entire organization is labeled a "no-smoking" zone. This places the onus on smokers to find an appropriate place to light up, rather than on nonsmokers to go out of their way to find clean air.
- Policies that ban smoking throughout the organization. In the view of smokers this is an extreme solution, but a handful of firms bar employees from smoking on the

premises. Top-level management enthusiasm is required to enact this restriction.

- Policies that preclude the hiring of smokers. Now given the legal stamp of approval, these sweeping policies are justified on the grounds that employees who smoke are likely to be sicker, miss more days of work, or be less productive than nonsmokers.

The aggressive participation of at least one high-level manager in planning and implementing new smoking policies is vital. At a minimum, that individual must

- Work actively to garner support from other top managers.
- Set aside time for hands-on participation in the development of a well-thought-out rationale and policy.
- Make certain the program includes information, education, and the opportunity and incentive for employees to quit smoking.
- Ensure employee involvement and union representation at all appropriate levels.
- Make visible public appearances and statements about the new policies to top and middle management and to employees, families, retirees, trustees, and stockholders.
- Provide for a phase-in period rather than impose a new policy suddenly.

EMPLOYER LIABILITY: A GROWING PRESSURE FOR CHANGE

For a final word on the importance of correcting workplace pollution, we turn to the lawyers. As evidence mounts that air and water quality problems have a direct and damaging impact on employee health, employers who fail to provide a safe workplace are being sued in greater numbers. "Injured plaintiffs are beginning to take the offensive: they are lobbying on the local, state, and federal levels for protective legislation, and in the absence of such legislation, they are suing for injuries allegedly caused by indoor air pollution," observes the attorney Laurence S. Kirsch in "Liability for Indoor Air Pollution in the Workplace," an exhaustive review of recent court decisions on the subject.

Just how vulnerable are employers to indoor pollution-related liability suits? Here's some background:

Workers' compensation, a form of federal no-fault insurance, was devised as an alternative to liability suits. Ironically, the law was intended to protect employers from the costly damages sometimes awarded in court, as well as to compensate employees for injuries sustained on the job. Over the years, coverage has been extended to workers who fall ill as a consequence of occupational hazards; awards linked to indoor pollution fall under this category.

Because workers' compensation ceilings are low, some employees still seek grounds for pursuing a complaint in court. When employees charge intentional misconduct, a greater offense than simple negligence, or fraudulent concealment of hazards, legal action is often allowed. For example, workers at a Cincinnati chemical company went to court, claiming their employer knew about hazardous fumes but maliciously failed to provide appropriate warnings. A similar suit was permitted against Johns-Manville when workers claimed the asbestos manufacturer hid information about the product's dangers.

According to Kirsch's review, liability suits linked to indoor pollution have been brought when the employee:

- Seeks an injunction to abate a pollution hazard rather than to be granted a monetary award.
- Challenges an unemployment compensation or disability decision, claiming that a complaint associated with workplace pollution was not fairly considered.
- Is discharged after complaining about indoor pollution problems.

- Claims that sensitivity to indoor pollutants is a handicap covered under the provisions of the Vocational Rehabilitation Act.
- Files an assault charge. This bizarre legal justification was used in one suit in which an employee reported that his boss lit up a cigar and said, "Bill, I know you claim to have an allergy to tobacco smoke and you have presented statements from your doctor stating this, but there is no law against smoking, so I'm going to smoke."

While workers' compensation remains the main avenue of redress for injured or ailing workers, liability suits are clearly on the rise. The prospect of bitter and potentially ruinous lawsuits is a powerful incentive for employers to take corrective actions against workplace hazards.

PART III:
PUBLIC
POLICY

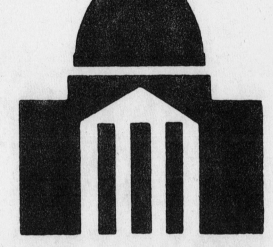

9
PRIVATE LIVES, PUBLIC RESPONSIBILITY
Forging Alliances for a Common Goal

While the environmental movements of the 1970s helped focus public and legislative attention on outdoor air and water pollution, no one has paid much heed to the indoor environment until very recently. Finally, though, there are some clear indications that the issue is being addressed. The EPA has put considerable energy into encouraging all Americans to have their homes tested for radon. Asbestos piping is being replaced in water systems where its deterioration has been noted, and the manufacture of most asbestos products will be phased out by 1997. Ordinances restricting indoor smoking in offices, restaurants, theaters, meeting places, and other public spaces have become commonplace. Knowledge about the proper use of building HVAC systems and how they can affect air quality has grown more sophisticated, making it easier to design, install, and maintain such systems properly. And numerous safer construction materials and relatively effective air and water purification systems have come onto the market.

These trends all reflect a greater awareness of indoor pollution problems and a growing commitment to mitigate them, but much more is needed. To improve the quality of indoor air and water where we live, work, and play, we first need more data about the sources and health effects of contaminants, the relationship between indoor air quality and energy conservation, and the best ways to mitigate the problems. Armed with these facts, concerned consumers and committed policymakers can then seek stronger statutes, more rigorously enforced contaminant standards, greater involvement from legislative and regulatory bodies, and the cooperation of the private sector.

Toward Consumer Activism

The best public policy changes are made by a broad consensus of affected players. Unfortunately, though, conflicting agendas often make such teamwork difficult.

For example, government representatives, industry leaders, environmental and consumer activists, and organized labor have distinct constituents to satisfy. Legislators with the authority to pass tough regulatory statutes are under pressure from a host of often-powerful special interests. While consumers and health experts may lobby for greater government protection, influential private sector companies generally favor deregulation, arguing that market forces should shape product availability. Building material manufacturers, home builders, chemical companies, and other industries are all likely to resist any legislation that adversely affects their pocketbooks. And employers have historically fought any measure to improve worker health and safety that results in increased costs.

How, then, can sound policies be established to safeguard the air we breathe and the water we drink both at home and at work? First and foremost, the public must *demand* that something be done. It will take sustained interest and a commitment to activism on the part of thousands, perhaps millions, of consumers to prod policymakers, product manufacturers, and building professionals into making needed changes.

Taking steps to protect your own family is only a beginning. Political action—lobbying, writing to your legislators, participating in organized protests, and donating funds to activist organizations—are all effective ways to become more deeply involved in the search for solutions to indoor pollution problems. Rather than viewing indoor residential pollution as a series of individual problems, homeowners and renters can join forces to demand safer products, more effective pollution mitigation techniques, and greater attention to their common concerns. Organizing at work, whether under the auspices of a labor union or informally through discussions with fellow employees, is similarly the best way to apply pressure to employers or building management personnel.

One fact is clear: Until the growing public concern about indoor air and water quality is translated into grassroots action, the nation's policymakers are unlikely to take the political risks necessary to change the status quo and improve the indoor environment.

Developing Standards: How Much Is Too Much?

Before we can effectively protect ourselves from unsafe exposure to contamination, we need to know just how much is safe. Yet there are no uniform air or water quality standards for residences in the United States, and existing workplace standards were developed primarily for industrial settings.

The contaminant standards that do exist are inconsistent and largely unenforceable. Most EPA standards were determined for outdoor air, where contaminants are more likely to be diluted, and are not appropriate to indoor spaces. The Occupational Safety and Health Administration's industrial guidelines are of dubious value in the home or in office buildings where increasing numbers of people work. In addition, OSHA figures are based on exposure to a range of contaminants by healthy workers in the mid-years of life who are on the job an average of forty hours a week. That's not very relevant to very young or very old people, who are often the most vulnerable to contaminants and likely to spend most of their time indoors. Nor do OSHA guidelines apply to people with respiratory problems, allergies, or other chemical sensitivities. They also ignore recent research that suggests low-level, chronic exposure to many toxic substances has a cumulative damaging effect.

The absence of reliable standards for indoor contaminants reflects in part the limitations of scientific knowledge. Right now, attempting to determine with certainty the health risks of indoor pollution is analogous to trying to balance your checkbook without knowing how much money you have deposited or how many checks you wrote. We simply don't know enough about all the risks.

Nonetheless, the limitations of understanding must not become an excuse to do nothing. According to Hal Levin, editor of the *Indoor Air Quality Update* newsletter, full implementation of the American Society of Heating, Refrigerating and Air-conditioning Engineers' ventilation standard for commercial buildings would eliminate up to 90 percent of any indoor air quality problems. Additional residential and workplace standards—both for single contaminants and for combinations of them—can be most efficiently developed if well-funded research into indoor air and water quality issues is given a higher priority within the scientific community and on the public agenda.

Ideally, compliance with any recommended standards will be voluntary—this eliminates the need for an unwieldy enforcement bureaucracy. However, if building system experts, product manufacturers, and industrial polluters prove unable or unwilling to police themselves, federal, state, and local authorities will have to step in with mandatory, and strictly enforced, standards. After all, the health and safety of the American public is at stake.

RECOMMENDATIONS: THE PUBLIC SECTOR

Lawmakers, public health experts, and others with influence on policy need to focus greater attention on indoor air and water quality issues because the problems won't go away if they are ignored. ''The ostrich effect doesn't help anyone," says Dr. Charlene W. Bayer, a research scientist at Georgia Tech Research Institute.

One important step is to provide public education. People are powerless to protect themselves against contaminants they have never been warned about. Readable, practical information about indoor pollution should be widely distributed. Richard J. Guimond, who directs the EPA's Office of Radiation Programs, emphasizes the importance of disseminating material written in nontechnical terms. "We need to do more than just throw brochures at the public. We should be presenting information in a way that they can understand," says Guimond.

Additional legislation may be necessary to improve the quality of the indoor environment. At the federal level, congressional hearings have already brought together experts in the public and private sectors and in the nation's leading academic institutions to help legislators make informed decisions. A major piece of federal legislation, the Indoor Air Quality Act, is being considered. When Congressman Joseph Kennedy II of Massachusetts introduced the bill in the House, he said:

Mr. Speaker, take a deep breath. The air that is now in your lungs passed through several hundred feet of dark, dusty, dirty ductwork before reaching this room. Twenty-seven species of fungus have been found growing in the dark recesses of building ventilation systems. Viruses and bacteria that thrive in air ducts have been proven to cause influenza, pneumonia, tuberculosis, and . . . deadly Legionnaire's disease.

Mr. Speaker, this is a problem that has remained hidden for too long in the dusty corners and dark bowels of the buildings around the country. I took off the grates in my own office . . . and found mildew, mold, and spores nearly two inches thick in the heating duct. If every one of our colleagues did the same, I don't think we would have any problem in passing this bill tomorrow.

The Indoor Air Quality Act, which was simultaneously introduced in the Senate by George Mitchell of Maine, would establish an Office of Indoor Air Quality within the EPA and an interagency Council on Indoor Air Quality to coordinate the work of all involved federal agencies. The bill would also provide grant monies to state and local programs, encourage research, mandate the EPA to prepare health advisories on indoor air contaminants and a plan for reducing their concentration levels, improve the management of pollution problems in federal buildings, establish an information clearinghouse, and direct the National Institute for Occupational Safety and Health (NIOSH) to develop model strategies for assessing and mitigating contamination in sick buildings.

Passage of the Indoor Air Quality Act would be an invaluable tool to accomplish six recommendations:

1. Improve coordination of federal indoor pollution activities.
2. Encourage and fund scientific research.
3. Encourage widespread adoption of the ASHRAE standard.
4. Incorporate indoor air quality standards into building codes.
5. Extend and enforce water quality legislation.
6. Restrict smoking in public places.

Improve Coordination of Federal Indoor Pollution Activities
Responsibility for the quality of the indoor environment is highly fragmented, with sixteen different federal agencies responsible for various aspects of indoor pollution. Just a sampling of their activities:

• The Environmental Protection Agency, which was established in 1970 to consolidate federal environmental activities, has increased its involvement with indoor pollution, but the issue still represents only a fraction of the agency's budget. Radon mitigation and asbestos reduction have been particular priorities.

- The Department of Energy is responsible for energy conservation programs in new buildings and residences; it conducts basic research into the relationship between energy conservation and indoor pollution and health problems.
- The Bonneville Power Administration, an agency of the Department of Energy, was one of the first federal organizations to study residential air quality issues, especially the link between energy conservation and contaminant levels.
- The Occupational Safety and Health Administration and the National Institute for Occupational Safety and Health are involved in worker health and safety issues, including those linked to indoor air quality.
- The Consumer Product Safety Commission, which is authorized to remove unsafe products from the marketplace, has successfully banned asbestos-containing spackling compounds and has tried to bar the sale of urea-formaldehyde foam insulation.
- The Federal Trade Commission monitors the truth and accuracy of consumer advertising. It has moved, for example, to bar two air cleaner manufacturers from making misleading claims about their products.

While the work of each of these federal agencies is very valuable, the patchwork approach to research, contaminant standards, and policymaking is highly inefficient. Regulatory authority is divided, public information has to be obtained from scores of different sources, and costly duplication of services is inevitable. "Sixteen agencies meddling around . . . is a formula for disaster," says Senator John H. Chafee of Rhode Island.

RECOMMENDATION: Improve the coordination of federal government policymaking, research, and educational services. Whether the decision is made to centralize authority for indoor pollution within a single federal agency or to create a consortium of involved agencies to share information and resources and to prevent service overlaps, we cannot afford the splintered approach that exists today.

Encourage and Fund Scientific Research

Unless public policies are closely linked to sound scientific research, they are likely to toss haplessly in the winds of political conflict and controversy. "Policy and science are often decoupled," complains Susan Rose, who manages the Department of Energy's Radon Research Program. "Mechanisms to relink them are urgently needed." Unfortunately, scientific research is limited by the paucity of available governmental funds, making it hard to develop sound public policies.

Gauging the real-life hazards of most industrial products is like blind men trying to describe an elephant. For example, there are some 1,200 different types of carpet adhesives available on the market today, each of which emits a different combination of contaminants at levels that depend on the age, construction, and ventilation system of the building where they are used, as well as on the weather. Which of these adhesives should be tested and what should they be tested for? Should they be tested the day they are used, several weeks later, or after the most intense chemical outgassing is over, usually several months after the product is applied? How can scientists simulate the actual environment of a home or office in their laboratories? And in the meantime, what should be done when carpeting needs to be installed? We don't yet have clear scientific answers to these questions, but we do know that expanded testing is practical only if better instrumentation and relatively simple, inexpensive, and rapid measurement techniques are made available.

Along with improved testing, research that can serve as a foundation for good public policies needs to include more animal studies; comparisons between chronic, long-term contaminant exposure and acute, short-term exposure; a greater understanding of the synergistic effects of exposure to a multitude of contaminants at any level; epidemiological studies to determine who is most likely to become ill as a result of indoor pollution; and a better understanding of effective mitigation techniques.

RECOMMENDATION: Increase government funds for indoor air and water quality research. By allocating adequate resources, policymakers advance the cause of science, provide a sound underpinning for policymaking, and let manufacturers, building owners and operators, and the concerned public know that indoor pollution is a governmental priority.

Encourage Widespread Adoption of the ASHRAE Standard

In 1977 the American Society of Heating, Refrigeration and Air-conditioning Engineers published its first guideline to indoor ventilation in commercial buildings. The ASHRAE standard, revised in 1981 and again in 1989, is entirely voluntary, but it has become the bellwether for many state and local building codes and has been widely adopted by engineers and builders. Based on the assumption that it is impossible to please 100 percent of the people 100 percent of the time, ASHRAE defines its objective as maintaining a ventilation rate that provides air of an acceptable quality for 80 percent of a building's occupants. A further criterion is that the indoor air contain no contaminants at concentrations known to be harmful.

ASHRAE Standard 62-1989 states that for every building occupant, a minimum ventilation rate of 15 cubic feet per minute of fresh outdoor air must circulate through the building. In commercial buildings, this technical specification is almost always achieved through the HVAC system. The ventilation rate was designed with the objective of reducing carbon dioxide concentrations to an acceptable level; while carbon dioxide itself is not a health threat, its presence suggests that other, more toxic pollutants are also in the air. In addition, the new ASHRAE standard requires that appropriate documentation be furnished for HVAC systems and that the systems be easy to clean and maintain.

RECOMMENDATION: ASHRAE Standard 62-1989 should be routinely followed by engineers and builders and should be incorporated into state and local building codes. While the ASHRAE standard is not perfect—it is particularly weak in terms of regulating the concentrations of specific contaminants—it represents the most successful attempt to balance energy conservation with the health and safety of building occupants.

Incorporate Indoor Air Quality Standards into Building Codes

The first building code to be passed in the United States, enacted in 1867 in New York City as part of the New York Tenement Law, specified that every tenement building be equipped with ventilators, fire escapes, water closets, and garbage receptacles. In the years since, stricter state and local codes have become commonplace. Today, building codes specify how much insulation has to be used, how far apart wall studs can be placed, what type of foundation is appropriate, minimum window size, and countless other complex and sometimes arcane construction details. Together, these standards assure structural soundness and provide a minimum degree of protection to potential buyers of resident and commercial dwellings.

But very few codes take indoor air quality into consideration. By mandating ventilation standards, the use of safe construction materials, and limits on the concentration of known pollutants, building codes have the potential to be an effective tool for controlling pollution inside residential and commercial buildings.

RECOMMENDATION: Appropriate state and local agencies or legislative bodies should incorporate indoor air quality standards into their building codes and provide the funding and staff to see that those codes are enforced. Model building codes should be developed by professional associations and government agencies.

Extend and Enforce Water Quality Legislation

In an era when we can send probes into outer space and penetrate the hidden secrets of submolecular particles, providing pure drinking water sounds elementary. But while this country has done a better job than most, we are a long way from developing a dependable drinking water supply. These are the major policy problems:

- Enforcement of existing federal water quality standards has been lackadaisical at best. The National Wildlife Federation filed suit against the EPA in late 1988, saying that the agency's enforcement of the Safe Drinking Water Act was "virtually nonexistent." The suit claimed that although 101,588 violations of water quality standards had been documented by the EPA during the preceding year, only 50 enforcement actions were launched.
- The federal and local water quality legislation currently on the books does not fully safeguard household water. The American Water Works Association estimates that only 59,000 of the 210,000 community water systems in this country are governed by the Safe Drinking Water Act. Systems that are not in year-round use and those that serve fewer than 3,300 people are currently exempt.
- The funding to solve water quality problems has not been made available. Without adequate financial and technical support, water utilities, especially the smaller ones, cannot comply with increasingly strict standards.
- Local water utilities have taken a largely passive role in the struggle to improve drinking water. Rather than lobbying legislators to devote more resources to cleanup

efforts or encouraging their customers to install water filters in their homes and businesses, most water companies have concentrated on seeking exemptions from stricter standards.

RECOMMENDATION: The provision of safe drinking water must become a matter of highest priority to policymakers and environmental activists. Needed are:

- Adequate funding for state and federal agencies responsible for the enforcement of water quality standards.
- New laws that cover all community water systems.
- Financial and technical resources to help utilities and individuals upgrade their water systems and install new purification equipment.
- Incentives for community water systems to meet or exceed water quality standards. Experimentation with alternative treatment techniques, such as the use of specially constructed wetlands for water purification, should be encouraged.
- Adequate support for research into the toxicity of waterborne chemicals and purification techniques.

Restrict Smoking in Public Places

In recent years, smoking has lost much of its panache as a socially acceptable—indeed, socially desirable—habit. Despite intensive lobbying from the tobacco industry, the public clamor for restrictions on smoking has never been higher, particularly in light of findings that environmental tobacco smoke has grave health consequences for nonsmokers.

Action on Smoking and Health (ASH), a Washington, D.C., based nonprofit agency that works to reduce smoking in public places, reports that forty-four states have passed legislation with at least minimal restrictions on smoking in public places. Thirty-two states limit smoking in government offices, while nineteen impose restrictions on smoking in all work-places, both public and private. Only seven states—Alabama, Illinois, Missouri, North Carolina, Tennessee, Virginia, and Wyoming—have no statutes at all on smoking. In addition, many private employers have established no-smoking zones or segregated smoking and nonsmoking workers.

More regulations against smoking in public places are appropriate. As former Surgeon General C. Everett Koop has observed, "The choice to smoke cannot interfere with the nonsmokers' right to breathe air free of tobacco smoke. The right of smokers to smoke ends where their behavior affects the health and well-being of others." ASH has sued the Occupational Safety and Health Administration in U.S. District Court to ban or severely limit smoking in every workplace in the country. The Federal Aviation Administration has already banned smoking on domestic flights of six hours or less. The trend toward reducing, if not eliminating, smoking in most public places is clearly accelerating.

RECOMMENDATION: Given the known health effects of passive smoking, as well as the synergistic damage created when other contaminants are present, smokers should be segregated from nonsmokers at work and in other public places—or smoking should be banned altogether.

RECOMMENDATIONS: THE PRIVATE SECTOR

The private sector also has a significant role to play in improving indoor air and water quality. ASHRAE has taken the lead in urging that engineering and building systems professionals pay greater attention to indoor pollution problems. Other professional associations, as well as many labor unions, are following suit.

Greater responsiveness from product manufacturers is clearly called for. There are many ways to reduce the use of contaminating materials without significantly increasing manufacturing costs. Making the switch to formaldehyde-free glues in the production of wood products and furniture, for example, can be done with relative ease, especially if consumers make strategic use of their purchasing power. By making educated buys—and letting manufacturers know why a contaminant-free product was selected—homeowners, tenants, workers, and building designers can all influence manufacturing practices. "A safer product will be consumer-driven. They will demand a safe product and force companies to respond," says Dr. Charlene W. Bayer of Georgia Tech.

Dr. Michael Hodgson, director of the University of Pittsburgh's Occupational and Environmental Health Program, described the moral imperative that must be lodged within the private sector. "Private ownership carries social responsibility," said Hodgson, noting that this is constitutional law within certain European nations. "Shoddy work doesn't have a place in today's world." That means that manufacturers should create safe products, builders should design sound buildings, and managers should operate them in a manner that is consistent with the health of the occupants—even if profits fall slightly as a result.

Here are some other recommendations for expanding the private sector's role in improving the indoor environment.

Determine Where the Buck Stops

The decisions made by architects, contractors, engineers, and interior designers all have a major impact on the indoor air and water quality of commercial dwellings. But when it comes to shouldering responsibility for sick building syndrome or other health-related contamination problems, building professionals are usually more likely to point fingers than to declare "mea culpa."

Someone should be in charge of identifying and correcting indoor air and water quality problems as they arise. Harry S. Truman kept a sign on his desk that read, "The buck stops here," and that's what's needed in the building industry as well. One solution is to pay the design team of a commercial building to assume long-term responsibility for its operation. Experts have suggested, for example, that an architect receive a fee for ten years following building construction to monitor and, if necessary, to revise design specifications with the goal of maintaining healthy indoor air. This approach provides an incentive for architects to minimize contamination and plan for adequate ventilation during the design process. It also tells both tenants and employees who has final authority for correcting any problems that might arise.

RECOMMENDATION: Every commercial building should place one individual or a team of building system professionals in charge of correcting indoor air and water quality problems. A formal grievance procedure should be established to provide tenants and workers a way to lodge complaints and an assurance that they will be adequately addressed.

Certify Indoor Pollution Investigators

As the public becomes more aware of indoor pollution problems, test kits, mitigation devices, and contractor services are being heavily advertised around the country. Unfortunately, consumers have no way of gauging the qualifications or reliability of any individual or firm who offers to test for contamination or to eliminate it. Because indoor pollution is often invisible, the problem is complicated by the fact that a consumer often cannot tell whether a job has been done well, or at all. The enormous potential for fraud became particularly clear after the EPA recommended widespread radon testing. Suddenly, snake-oil salesmen were everywhere, peddling miracle cures and using outrageous scare tactics to persuade gullible homeowners to part with their money for unnecessary improvements.

The complete absence of formal licensing and accreditation procedures for people who call themselves indoor air

and water quality experts allows such abuse to go unchecked. A policy change is clearly needed. "If the person
who cuts my hair has to have a license, then the person who
controls the air that I breathe ought to have some certification," said Dr. James E. Woods, Jr., an expert in building
construction at Virginia Polytechnic Institute.

An accreditation procedure that establishes minimum
qualifications and requires continuing education and periodic
retesting could bring a cohesiveness and credibility that is
currently lacking in the field. A number of key decisions need
to be made, including whether the accreditation procedure
should be run by a professional association or a government
regulatory body and whether firms or individuals should
be accredited. It also will be crucial to develop a procedure
that does not reduce competition or exclude small business
owners.

A report on indoor air quality credentialing, prepared for
the Environmental Protection Agency ("Plan for Establishing
a Credentialing System for Individuals and/or Companies that
Investigate, Evaluate, and/or Mitigate Indoor Air Quality
Problems") by David A. Swankin states: "There is no obvious
right way to structure a voluntary certification system for
indoor air quality investigators and mitigators. What is right
is what is acceptable: to those who provide these services; to
those who utilize these services; and to those with an interest
in improving indoor air quality."

Swankin says a viable accreditation procedure must

- "be acceptable to all of the interested parties, including members of the profession, the building community, building product manufacturers, the real estate
  sales and financing communities, public health officials
  and consumers.
- "be based on an ability to differentiate between those
  who possess demonstrable minimum knowledge of indoor air quality investigation and mitigation skills and
  those who do not.
- "be flexible enough to accommodate any pollutant-

specific certification systems currently in place or enacted in the future.

- "become self-supporting in as short a time frame as
possible."

RECOMMENDATION: Develop an accreditation system for
individuals who investigate and mitigate indoor air and water
quality problems with an eye toward protecting the public
from fraudulent practices while enhancing the professional-
ism of the investigators. As Harry Rector, a research scientist
with GEOMET Technologies, said, the objective of certification is "to see whether this person can be turned loose to use
his judgment."

Educate and Support Building System Professionals

The expertise of interior designers, architects, contractors, and engineers can be channeled into improving the indoor environment at home and in the workplace—so long as
these professionals have state-of-the-art knowledge of their
own fields. Yet despite the proliferation of specialized jour-
nals in so many other fields, not one is dedicated exclusively
to the study of indoor pollution. And while a number of professional associations have taken an interest in the subject,
there has been little effort to coordinate educational programs or to agree on policy recommendations.

Along with the difficulties of remaining current in a field
where knowledge is expanding rapidly, building owners and
operators are fearful of being asked to shoulder extra financial burdens for pollution mitigation. Inevitably, this creates
resistance to acknowledging and confronting indoor air and
water quality problems. If building professionals are to contribute their expertise, they first need assurance that mitigation is a cooperative enterprise and that responsibilities will
be fairly distributed.

RECOMMENDATION: Technical information should be dis-
seminated as widely as possible, via private and government-

sponsored conferences and publications, to professionals in the building trades. In addition, professional associations and public agencies should cooperate in making available the technical, legal, and financial assistance that building owners and operators need to solve indoor pollution problems.

GOOD PUBLIC POLICY: AN ALTERNATIVE TO LITIGATION

A recent Illinois court ruling allows prosecutors to file criminal negligence charges against businesses believed to have caused harm to their employees as a result of contaminated indoor air. This decision is expected to spawn a wave of suits charging that the use of faulty ventilation systems constitutes a failure to protect employee health.

But are lawsuits the best way to eliminate indoor pollution in commercial buildings? Laurence S. Kirsch, the Washington, D.C., attorney, thinks not, noting that suits are costly and time-consuming and often fail to satisfy either the employee or the employer. In "Liability for Indoor Air Pollution in the Workplace," a report on recent litigation in the field, Kirsch observes that no monetary settlement can adequately compensate a worker for injury or illness and that the capriciousness of settlements does not allow the defendant or the plaintiff to predict the outcome of any suit with assurance.

Far better, urges Kirsch and many other responsible policymakers, to address the concerns that ultimately give rise to lawsuits. "The key to the resolution of indoor air pollution liability is guidance," writes Kirsch. "Guidance to individuals about the risks posed by indoor air pollution; guidance to employers, building owners, and the broader group of actors who play a role in building design and specification; guidance to the state and local governments who may wish to make decisions concerning building codes or product specifications; and guidance to the federal government which, when faced with additional data, may decide that indoor air pollution requires mandatory federal action. The provision of such guidance would do immeasurably more to alleviate indoor air quality problems than could the common law system at its best.''

Kirsch believes such a system would effectively serve all concerned parties. He writes: ''The commercial and industrial community would be given precisely what it now lacks: a simple goal that can be satisfied at a known cost. Industries would have an incentive to adhere to the standards because such adherence may obviate the more dreaded and unpredictable random strike lawsuits; moreover, adherence to the standards might constitute evidence of a company's due care and good faith. In turn, employees would achieve their goal: a safer workplace.''

Today, the public is waking up to the very real hazards contained in the air we breathe and the water we drink, both at home and at work. But the indoor pollution problem need not become a field day for litigators. Cooperation, not confrontation, should be the order of the day. Organized and politically active consumers willing to exercise their enormous clout can forge strong links with responsive public and private sectors. Together all Americans can take the steps necessary to make the indoor environment a safe and healthy one.

Appendix

FEDERAL AIR AND WATER LEGISLATION

The following laws have helped to improve air and water quality in the United States. Initially prompted by concerns about the outdoor environment, most of this legislation has had a positive impact on indoor pollution as well.

Key Laws

- The Clean Air Act of 1970 was an ambitious piece of legislation and had the goal of improving the quality of America's air to the point that inhaling it would pose no health risk. Although residents of nearly every city breathe easier today because of the act, the zero-emission goal has remained far out of reach. The act, which is enforced by the EPA, is expected to be renewed in 1991.
- The Clean Water Act of 1972, the first pathbreaking piece of federal water legislation, spelled out the nation's commitment to "restore and maintain the chemical, physical and biological integrity of the nation's waters." Under the law, which is enforced by the EPA, all states are mandated to adopt specific water quality standards for every stream within their borders. Industrial and municipal waste discharges are strictly regulated and wetlands are protected. The Water Quality Act of 1987 reauthorized and strengthened the Clean Water Act.
- The Safe Drinking Water Act of 1974 requires the EPA to set limits for water pollutants so that "no known or

anticipated effects on the health of persons occur.''
State governments have the primary responsibility for
enforcing the limits, called maximum contaminant levels (MCLs). Amendments in 1977 extended technical
assistance and provided grants to the states; 1986
amendments strengthened the protection of wellheads
and aquifers.

Asbestos

- The Asbestos Information Act requires manufacturers
  to provide the EPA with specifications on asbestos
  products that have been manufactured in the past so
  that the agency can become an information clearinghouse.
- The Consumer Product Safety Act and the Hazardous
  Substances Act allow the Consumer Product Safety
  Commission to establish safety standards for products
  containing asbestos and to institute recalls or bans as
  appropriate.
- The General Industry Standard and the Construction
  Standard, promulgated by the Occupational Safety and
  Health Administration, determine safety thresholds for
  airborne concentrations of asbestos fibers.
- The National Emission Standards for Hazardous Air
  Pollutants, enforced by the EPA, establishes standards
  for demolition, and renovation projects and procedures
  for asbestos emission control.
- The Asbestos Hazard Emergency Response Act of 1986
  requires the EPA to develop a system under which all
  school buildings are inspected for asbestos and appropriate responses taken.
- The Safe Drinking Water Act requires annual testing of
  municipal water supplies to detect the concentration
  levels of asbestos.
- The Clean Water Act of 1972 establishes standards for
  facilities that discharge asbestos into public sewers or
  navigable waters.

- The Hazardous Materials Transportation Act, enforced by the Department of Transportation, regulates the conditions under which asbestos may be transported.

Radon

- The Indoor Radon Abatement Act of 1988 was passed in the fall of 1988 as an amendment to the Toxic Substances Control Act of 1976. It authorizes $45 million to be spent over a three-year period for radon-related activities at the state and federal levels. The act also establishes a long-term goal of reducing indoor radon levels to those typically found outdoors, approximately 0.2 Ci/L, and provides funds for the states to assist in the development of radon assessment and mitigation programs.

Lead

- The Lead Contamination Control Act of 1988 bans lead-lined water coolers (which is especially important in the schools, where they have been in widespread use). The act also expands a lead-screening program for children and directs the EPA to assist schools in testing their facilities for lead.
- The Lead-Based Paint Act of 1971 prohibits the use of paint with lead pigment in federally financed construction.
- The Clean Air Act of 1970 called for new automobiles to run on lead-free fuel—critical since 95 percent of airborne lead that belched from vehicles at the time. Currently only one-tenth of a gram of lead is allowed in each gallon of gas.
- The Safe Drinking Water Act of 1986 bans the use of lead-based solder in plumbing systems.

Environmental Pollutants

- The Resource Conservation and Recovery Act of 1976 focuses on the transport, storage, treatment, and disposal of hazardous materials, and gives the EPA power to protect water and air from contamination. Congress renewed the act in 1984, adding a program to clean up leaking underground storage tanks.

- The Comprehensive Environmental Response, Compensation and Liability Act of 1980 (CERCLA), better known as the Superfund, provides funds to clean up hazardous waste sites, including those that threaten air or water quality. Congress passed the $9 billion Superfund Amendments and Reauthorization Act (SARA) in 1986, giving state agencies authority to prosecute owners of toxic waste dumps that pollute air, soil, or water. The legislation is enforced by the EPA.

- The Federal Insecticide, Fungicide and Rodenticide Act of 1972 was intended to ensure that pesticides marketed in this country don't threaten the public health or the environment. The act gave the EPA authority to test and regulate pesticides to prevent the contamination of air and water with dangerous chemicals. Efforts to strengthen the measure have been under way for well over a decade, but a deadlock between Congress, industry, and environmentalists has so far prevented new legislation.

- The Toxic Substances Control Act of 1976 gave the EPA authority to require testing of new chemicals before they can be put on the market.

- The Federal Hazardous Substances Act, passed in the fall of 1988, requires manufacturers to label hazardous art materials according to the standards recommended by the American Society for Testing and Materials.

- Right-to-know laws require employers to inform workers about the risks associated with specific toxic substances. To date, however, the low concentrations of pollutants associated with indoor air quality problems have rarely been covered under this legislation.

ORGANIZATIONS INVOLVED WITH INDOOR POLLUTION

FEDERAL AGENCIES

Environmental Protection Agency

Established in December 1970 to consolidate federal environmental activities, the EPA is authorized to deal with air and water pollution, pesticides, the disposal of municipal and hazardous wastes, and radiation. Indoor pollution represents only a small portion of the agency's efforts, but radon mitigation and asbestos reduction have been particular priorities. In addition to its headquarters in Washington, D.C., the EPA has ten regional offices covering every state in the union.

Further information: Public Information Center, 820 Quincy St., N.W., Washington, D.C. 20011. (202) 829-3535.

EPA publications can be ordered from: 401 M St., S.W., Washington, D.C. 20460. (202) 382-4355.

The EPA maintains several information hotlines:

- *Asbestos Information Line.* (800) 835-6700
- *Radon Test Information.* (800) 767-7236
- *Superfund Hotline.* (800) 424-9346. (202) 382-3000 in Washington, D.C.
- *Safe Drinking Water Act Hotline.* (800) 426-4791. (202) 382-5533 in Washington, D.C.
- *National Pesticides Telecommunications Network.* (800) 858-PEST. (806) 743-3091 in Texas.
- *Toxic Substances Control Act Information Service.* (202) 554-1404.

Department of Energy

The Department of Energy is responsible for energy conservation programs in new buildings and residences. It also conducts basic research into the relationship between energy conservation and indoor pollution and health problems. Six DOE agencies are active in the area of indoor air quality:

Bonneville Power Administration has been involved with indoor pollution since 1980, when it began to evaluate the environmental effects of residential weatherization. It continues to study the link between energy conservation and contaminant levels and provides detailed, well-illustrated booklets to residential homeowners, builders, and utilities.

Further information: Public Involvement Office, Bonneville Power Administration, Box 12999, Portland, Ore. 97212. (503) 230-3478. (800) 624-9495 in Washington, Idaho, Montana, Utah, Nebraska, and California. (800) 841-5867 in Oregon.

Tennessee Valley Authority cooperates with the Bonneville Power Administration and federal laboratories to develop energy conservation programs and strategies for dealing with the poor indoor air quality often found in tight homes.

Further information: Tennessee Valley Authority, 400 West Summit Hill Dr., Knoxville, Tenn. 37902. (800) 251-9242. (800) 362-9250 in Tennessee.

Office of Conservation and Renewable Energy focuses on the relationship between air exchange rates and indoor air quality; how indoor air is affected by outdoor contaminants, such as radon, by human activities, and by building materials; and the development of appropriate measurement and control techniques.

Further information: Conservation and Renewable Energy Inquiry and Referral Service, Box 8900, Silver Spring, Md. 20907. (800) 523-2929.

Office of Environment, Safety, and Health distributes information on indoor air quality, supports research, reviews legislation and other efforts to implement indoor air quality policy, and conducts aerial surveillance to identify regions with high radiation levels.

Further information: Office of Environment Safety and Health, 1000 Independence Ave., S.W., Washington, D.C. 20585. (202) 586-6151.

Office of Energy Research is research-oriented and focuses on the risks associated with indoor radon as part of its larger mandate to study all types of ionizing radiation.

Further information: Office of Energy Research, 1000 Independence Ave., S.W., Washington, D.C. 20585. (202) 586-5430.

Office of Nuclear Energy is involved with specific remedial programs, including efforts to lower indoor radon levels in regions of uranium disposal.

Further information: Office of Nuclear Energy, 1000 Independence Ave., S.W., Washington, D.C. 20585. (202) 586-6450.

Consumer Product Safety Commission

Established as an independent agency by the 1972 Consumer Product Safety Act, the commission works with industry to develop voluntary product safety standards. It can also institute mandatory standards or ban products altogether and has been involved in efforts to restrict the sale of some asbestos products and urea-formaldehyde foam insulation.

Further information: Office of the Secretary, Consumer Product Safety Commission, 5401 Westbard Ave., Bethesda, Md. 20207. (800) 638-2772.

Occupational Safety and Health Administration

The Occupational Safety and Health Act of 1970 established the Occupational Safety and Health Administration under the Department of Labor. OSHA establishes and enforces workplace health and safety standards, concentrating primarily on air quality in factories rather than in offices.

Further information: Occupational Safety and Health Administration, 200 Constitution Ave., N.W., Washington, D.C. 20210. (800) 582-1708. (202) 523-8148 in Washington, D.C.

Department of Housing and Urban Development
The Department of Housing and Urban Development issues Minimum Property Standards, which specify standards for radiation and ventilation in government-financed housing through HUD, the Farmers' Home Administration, and the Veterans Administration. The HUD Office of Manufactured Housing Standards limits formaldehyde emissions of particle-board and plywood paneling. Publications on formaldehyde are available.

Further information: Department of Housing and Urban Development, 451 7th St., S.W., Washington, D.C. 20410. (202) 755-6420.

Farmers' Home Administration, 14th St. and Independence Ave., S.W., Washington, D.C. 20410. (202) 447-6903.

Veterans Administration, Office of Public Affairs, 810 Vermont Ave., N.W., Washington, D.C. 20420. (202) 233-2300.

Health and Human Services
The following agencies of the Department of Health and Human Services, which is charged with preserving the public health, are engaged in some indoor pollution activities:

National Institute for Occupational Safety and Health, a part of the Centers for Disease Control, will respond to requests to conduct comprehensive indoor air quality investigations in commercial buildings and to make recommendations for improvements.

Further information: Hazard Evaluations and Technical Assistance Branch, 4676 Columbia Pkwy., Cincinnati, Ohio 45226. (800) 356-4674. (513) 841-4374 in Ohio.

National Toxicology Program, a part of the National Institutes of Health, compiles information about the health effects of toxic chemicals.

Further information: National Toxicology Program, P.O. Box 12233, Research Triangle Park, N.C. 27709. (919) 541-3991.

Food and Drug Administration regulates foods, drugs, and cosmetics that may pose a threat to public health and under some circumstances can pollute indoor air. In particular, products in aerosol cans can be a problem.

Further information: Food and Drug Administration, 5600 Fishers Ln., Rockville, Md. 20857. (301) 443-3170.

Office on Smoking and Health, a part of the Centers for Disease Control, operates a Technical Information Center, which provides scientific information about smoking.

Further information: Office on Smoking and Health, Center for Health Promotion and Education, Parklawn Building, Room 1-10, 5600 Fishers Ln., Rockville, Md. 20857.

National Library of Medicine manages the MEDLAR on-line system, which contains data on the toxicity of chemicals to humans and animals.

Further information: MEDLAR—Management Section, National Library of Medicine, 8600 Rockville Pike, Bethesda, Md. 20209.

Other Federal Agencies
Federal Aviation Administration monitors air quality in airplanes.

Further information: Federal Aviation Administration, 800 Independence Ave., S.W., Washington, D.C. (202) 366-4000.

Interstate Commerce Commission regulates smoking on interstate buses and intercity passenger trains.

Further information: Interstate Commerce Commission, 12th St. and Constitution Ave., N.W., Washington, D.C. 20423. (202) 275-7119.

Federal Trade Commission monitors the truth and accuracy of consumer advertising and has halted air cleaner manufacturers from making misleading claims about their products.

Further information: Federal Trade Commission, Pennsylvania Ave. at 6th St., N.W., Washington, D.C. (202) 326-2222.

Government Accounting Office investigates the effectiveness of environmental regulations. A publications catalog is available.

Further information: Government Accounting Office, Box 6015, Gaithersburg, Md. 20877. (202) 275-2265.

Office of Technology Assessment, the investigative arm of Congress, looks into the operation of environmental programs mandated by federal laws and issues reports on them.

Further information: Office of Technology Assessment, 600 Pennsylvania Ave., S.E., Washington, D.C. 20510. (202) 224-8996.

STATE AGENCIES

The Environmental Protection Agency's "Directory of State Indoor Air Contacts" is by far the best source of information about agencies and individuals working on indoor air quality at the state level. The publication pulls together contact names and addresses in all fifty states on sixteen issues: asbestos; biologicals; building complaint investigations; combustion devices and gases; formaldehyde; health complaints; insulation; odors; paints, cleaners, and solvents; particulates; pesticides; radon; termiticides and chlordane; tobacco smoke; ventilation; and wood preservatives. "Directory of State Indoor Air Contacts" was prepared for the EPA by the Washington, D.C.–based Public Health Foundation.

Further information: EPA, 401 M St., S.W., Washington, D.C. 20460.

PRIVATE AND NOT-FOR-PROFIT AGENCIES

Action on Smoking and Health
2013 H St., N.W.
Washington, D.C. 20006
Publishes materials warning about the health hazards of
smoking to both smokers and nonsmokers and lobbies for
more restrictive anti-smoking legislation.

American Conference of Governmental Industrial Hygienists
6500 Glenway Ave., Building D-7
Cincinnati, Ohio 45211
(513) 661-7881
Focuses on the administrative and technical aspects of
worker health. Publishes "Threshold Limit Values of Airborne Contaminants," a regularly updated listing of contaminants commonly found in the workplace.

American Industrial Hygiene Association
475 Wolf Ledges Pkwy.
Akron, Ohio 44311
Maintains a list of industrial hygiene consultants who can
provide on-site technical assistance to employees or employers concerned about pollution in the workplace.

American Institute of Architects
1735 New York Ave., N.W.
Washington, D.C. 20006
(202) 626-7300
Conducts research on ventilation and indoor air quality.

American Lung Association
1740 Broadway
New York, N.Y. 10019
(212) 315-8700
Provides information on the health effects of indoor air
pollution. Offices are located in every state or contact the
national office listed here.

American Society of Heating, Refrigeration and
Air-conditioning Engineers
    1791 Tullie Circle, N.E.
    Atlanta, Ga. 30329
    (404) 636-8400
    Establishes standards for the design and operation
    of heating and cooling systems, including standards for
    ventilation. State and local governments use ASHRAE's
    standards as a model for building codes. Extensive publi-
    cations list available.

American Society for Testing and Materials
    1916 Race St.
    Philadelphia, Pa. 19103
    (215) 299-5400
    Establishes testing procedures and standards for airborne
    contaminants under the mandate of the Federal Hazard-
    ous Substances Control Act.

Americans for Non-Smokers' Rights
    2054 University Ave., Suite 500
    Berkeley, Calif. 94704
    (415) 841-3032
    Advocates for restrictive smoking policies in public places.

Asbestos Victims of America
    P.O. Box 559
    Capitola, Calif. 95010
    (408) 476-3646
    Provides information on the health effects and sources of
    asbestos and support for the victims of asbestos poison-
    ing.

Building Officials and Code Administrators International
    4051 West Flossmoor Rd.
    Country Club Hills, Ill. 48106
    (312) 799-2300
    Publishes a building code with ventilation standards and

building materials specifications that is widely used in the northeastern states.

Business Council on Indoor Air
1225 19th St., N.W., Suite 300
Washington, D.C. 20036
(202) 775-5887
Represents a wide spectrum of industries interested in indoor air quality, including engineers and manufacturers of chemicals, consumer products, and building materials.

Center for Safety in the Arts
5 Beekman St.
New York, N.Y. 10038
(212) 227-6220
Advocates for the safe manufacture and use of artist and hobby materials. Extensive publications are available.

Center for Science in the Public Interest
1755 S St., N.W.
Washington, D.C. 20009
(202) 332-9110
Conducts research and publishes information about toxic substances and other environmental issues.

Chemical Manufacturers Association
2501 M St., N.W.
Washington, D.C. 20037
(800) 262-8200
Operates a Chemical Referral Center to provide health and safety information about chemicals and chemical products. Open weekdays.

Citizens' Clearinghouse for Hazardous Waste
Box 926
Arlington, Va. 22216
(703) 276-7070
Established to disseminate information about toxic wastes

and their health effects and to help local citizens' groups organize to stop air and water pollution in their neighborhoods.

Environmental Defense Fund
1616 P St., N.W.
Washington, D.C. 20036
(202) 745-4879
Provides information on air and water quality legislation and the politics behind the laws. Orchestrated the successful suit to have DDT banned in the early 1970s.

Formaldehyde Institute
1330 Connecticut Ave., N.W.
Washington, D.C. 20036
(202) 659-0060
A trade association of makers and users of formaldehyde resins, the institute provides information on formaldehyde in consumer products.

GSX Chemical Services
Box 210799
Columbia, S.C. 29221
(800) 845-1019
Provides help in organizing community hazardous waste collection programs.

Hardwood Plywood Manufacturers Association
1825 Michael Faraday Dr.
Reston, Va. 22090
(703) 435-2900
Trade association that provides information on the use of formaldehyde-based glues in plywood products manufactured by its members.

Human Ecology Action League
P.O. Box 66637
Chicago, Ill. 60666
(312) 665-6575

A nonprofit, volunteer organization that disseminates information about environmental health issues through its chapters and affiliated support groups located throughout the country.

International Conference of Building Officials
5360 South Workman Mill Rd.
Whittier, Calif. 90601
(213) 699-0541
Publishes the *Uniform Building Code*, which is widely used in the north central and western states and includes standards for ventilation and building material specifications.

National Association of Home Builders (NAHB)
National Research Center
400 Prince Georges Blvd.
Upper Marlboro, Md. 20772
(301) 249-4000
A clearinghouse for information on indoor air quality.

National Appropriate Technology Assistance Service
Box 2525
Butte, Mont. 59702
(800) 428-2525
(800) 428-1718 in Montana
Answers questions about energy conservation, renewable energy, and indoor air quality.

National Asthma Center
National Jewish Hospital for Immunology and Respiratory Medicine
3800 East Colfax Ave.
Denver, Colo. 80206
(800) 222-5864 or (303) 388-4461
The center conducts research on respiratory disease and provides information through the "Lungline" telephone service.

National Center for Environmental Health Strategies
1100 Rural Ave.
Voorhees, N.J. 08043
(609) 429-5358
Provides informational, educational, and advocacy services to the public on chemical and environmental pollutants, with particular emphasis on the indoor environment. Publishes "The Delicate Balance" newsletter.

National Environmental Balancing Bureau
8224 Old Courthouse Rd.
Vienna, Va. 22180
Maintains a list of certified engineering firms that can provide on-site technical assistance to employees or employers concerned about pollution in the workplace.

National Foundation for the Chemically Hypersensitive
P.O. Box 9
Wrightsville Beach, N.C. 28480
(919) 256-5391
Provides information about the health effects of indoor air pollution.

National Research Council/National Academy of Sciences
2101 Constitution Ave., N.W.
Washington, D.C. 20418
(202) 334-2000
Conducts research on contaminant toxicity and testing procedures in the workplace.

Natural Resources Defense Council
40 West 20th St.
New York, N.Y. 10168
(212) 949-0049
Conducts research and initiates litigation intended to

improve household air quality while minimizing energy use.

Southern Building Code Conference
900 Montclair Rd.
Birmingham, Ala. 35213
(205) 591-1853
Publishes a building code that includes standards for ventilation and building materials. Has state and local government representation from twenty-five states.

WATER POLLUTION

American Water Resources Association
5410 Grosvenor Ln., Suite 220
Bethesda, Md. 20814
(301) 493-8600
Professional association of scientists, engineers, and water-related businesses that also publishes information of interest to the general public.

Association of State Water Quality Administrators
1911 Fort Meyer Dr., Suite 803
Arlington, Va. 22209
(703) 524-2428
Publishes information about the Safe Drinking Water Act and the states' administration of water quality programs.

Clean Water Fund
317 Pennsylvania Ave., S.E., Suite 200
Washington, D. C. 20003
(202) 547-2312
Conducts research and offers education programs at the national, state, and local levels for safe drinking water, control of toxic chemicals and solid waste, and protection of natural resources.

International Bottled Water Association
    113 North Henry St.
    Alexandria, Va. 22314
    (703) 683-5213
    Concerned about the quality and marketing of bottled water.

National Water Well Association
    P.O. Box 16737
    Columbus, Ohio 43216
    (614) 761-1777
    Provides publications about groundwater and wells.

Water Pollution Control Federation
    601 Wythe St.
    Alexandria, Va. 22314
    (703) 684-2400
    An association of companies and individuals interested in the political and technical aspects of water pollution with local affiliates in most states. The federation focuses on the treatment of municipal and industrial waste water.

Water Quality Association
    4151 Naperville Rd.
    Lisle, Ill. 60532
    (312) 369-1600
    An association of water purification equipment dealers and manufacturers that conducts water quality research and supplies information to the public.

SAMPLE LETTER TO A LEGISLATOR

Congressman Donald Dinglehousen
Cannon House Office Building
Washington, D.C. 20013

Dear Representative Dinglehousen,

I am writing to urge that you initiate or support federal legislation that will improve the quality of indoor air. As a consumer and a worker—as well as a voter—I am disturbed that so little effort has been made to pass laws to reduce pollution at home and in the workplace. Innovation in this area is sorely needed.

It has already been well established that polluted indoor air poses a serious threat to many Americans:

- The Environmental Protection Agency estimates that indoor pollution costs U.S. businesses *tens of billions* of dollars a year. Employee sick days, lost earnings, medical care, and diminished productivity all contribute to this staggering bill.
- The Consumer Product Safety Commission has identified 150 toxic chemicals commonly found in indoor air. The chemicals have been linked to cancer, allergies, birth defects, and psychological abnormalities.
- The World Health Organization estimates that up to 30 percent of new and remodeled office buildings cause symptoms associated with sick building syndrome.
- Toxic gases, virulent organisms, including those responsible for Legionnaire's disease, and pollens have been recorded indoors at levels far higher than those typically found outside.

Several measures should be addressed as part of any federal legislation on indoor air pollution:

- Toxins emitted by building materials, household cleaners, and cosmetics should be strictly regulated.
- States and cities should be encouraged to adopt ventilation standards at least as stringent as those set forth in the ASHRAE Standard 62-1989.
- More money should be made available to enforce existing workplace air quality standards and to develop strict new standards for offices.
- Smoking bans should be extended to all forms of public transportation, and airplane, bus, and train operators should be required to provide adequate fresh air.

Please keep me informed about your activities in the critical area of indoor pollution.

Sincerely,

An American Taxpayer

TESTING EQUIPMENT AND LABORATORIES

The Consumer Product Safety Commission can provide lists of local laboratories that will test for a range of contaminants as well as names of asbestos-control contractors. For further information contact: Office of the Secretary, Consumer Product Safety Commission, 5401 Westbard Ave., Bethesda, Md. 20207. (800) 638-2772.

The Environmental Protection Agency's Toxic Substances Control Act's Assistance Office also maintains lists of noncommercial labs that have been accredited by the agency. For further information contact: (202) 544-1404.

Branch offices of the EPA can provide names of asbestos-testing labs in your area. For referrals, call the Asbestos Information Line at (800) 835-6700.

Other sources of testing equipment and laboratories that evaluate test results are listed below. You may also want to check local Yellow Pages and state environmental health agencies for additional recommendations.

Radon Test Kits

Air Chek, Inc.
180 Glenn Bridge Rd.
Box 2000
Arden, N.C. 28704
(800) 257-2366
(704) 684-0893 in
North Carolina

American Radon
Corporation
8300 North Hayden Rd.
Suite 100
Scottsdale, Ariz. 85258
(602) 967-8029

American Radon
Consultants
3282 Chalfont Rd.
Shaker Heights, Ohio 44120
(216) 921-8398

Applied Technical Services
1190 Atlanta Industrial Dr.
Marietta, Ga. 30066
(800) 451-3405
(404) 423-1400 in Georgia

Honeywell, Inc.
1985 Douglas Dr., N.
Golden Valley, MN 55422
(612) 542-6723

Key Technology
P.O. Box 562
Jonestown, Pa. 17038
(717) 274-8310

National Draeger
Box 120
Pittsburgh, Pa. 15230
(412) 787-8383
FAX: (412) 787-2207

Nuclear Associates
100 Voice Rd.
Carle Place, N.Y. 11514
(516) 741-6360

Radon Analytical
Laboratories
8935 North Meridian St.
Suite 110
Indianapolis, Ind. 46260
(317) 843-0788

Radon Detection Services
Old York Rd.
Ringoes, N.J. 08551
(201) 788-3080

Radon Testing Corporation
of America
50 South Buchout
Irvington, N.Y. 10533
(800) 457-2366
(800) 537-7822 in New York

Scientific Analysis, Inc.
6012 East Shirley Ln.
Montgomery, Ala. 36117
(800) 345-2575
(800) 288-1580 in Alabama

Tech/Ops Landauer
2 Science Rd.
Glenwood, Ill. 60425
(312) 755-7911

Air-Testing Services and Equipment

BCM Engineers, Inc.
One Plymouth Meeting
Suite 506
Plymouth Meeting, Pa.
19462
(215) 825-3800
FAX: (215) 834-8236

Chem-Safe Laboratories
Box 546
Pullman, Wash. 99163
(509) 334-0922

Electro-Analytical
Laboratories
7118 Industrial Park Blvd.
Mentor, Ohio 44060
(216) 951-3514

Environmental Testing and
Technology
Box 369
Encinatas, Calif. 92024
(619) 436-5990

Lancaster Laboratories
2425 New Holland Pike
Lancaster, Pa. 17601
(717) 656-2301

RK Occupational and
Environmental Analysis
616 Warren St.
Alpha, N.J. 08865
(201) 454-6316

Safe Environments
Home and Office
Testing Laboratories
Box 489
San Leandro, Calif. 94577
(415) 843-6042
FAX: (415) 635-6730

Asbestos-Testing Laboratories

Alternative Ways
100 Essex Ave.
Bellmawr, N.J. 08031
(800) 547-0101

Building Environmental
Systems
3501 North MacArthur,
Suite 400B
Irving, Tex. 75062
(800) 982-0030
(214) 257-0787 in Texas

Laboratory Testing Services
75 Urban Ave.
Westbury, N.Y. 11590
(800) 433-0008

Source Finders Information
P.O. Box 758
Mt. Laurel, N.J. 08054
(609) 482-1151

Formaldehyde-Testing Laboratories

Air Quality Research
901 Grayson St.
Berkeley, Calif. 94710
(415) 644-2097

Assay Technology
1070 East Meadow Circle
Palo Alto, Calif. 94330
(800) 833-1258
(415) 424-9947

Crystal Diagnostics
30 Commerce Way
Woburn, Mass. 01801
(617) 933-4114

3M
Occupational Health and
Environmental Safety
Division
3M Center, Bldg. 220-3E-04
St. Paul, Minn. 55144
(612) 733-6486

Carbon Monoxide Detectors

Assay Technology
1070 East Meadow Circle
Palo Alto, Calif. 94330
(800) 833-1258
(415) 424-9947

Blue Sky Testing Labs
8655 39th Ave. S.
Seattle, Wash. 98118
(206) 721-2583

Lab Safety Supply
Box 1368
Janesville, Wis. 53547
(800) 356-0783

Neotronics N.A.
2144 Hilton Drive, N.W.
Gainsville, Ga. 30503
(800) 535-0606
(404) 535-0600 in Georgia
FAX: (404) 532-9282

Quantum Group, Inc.
Box 210347
San Diego, Calif. 92121
(800) 432-5599
(619) 457-3048 in California

Sensidyne
12345 Starkey Rd.
Largo, Fla. 34643
(800) 451-9444
(813) 530-3602 in Florida
FAX: (813) 539-0050

Water-Testing Laboratories

The following private laboratories can evaluate tap water in private residences:

Brown and Caldwell Laboratories   (415) 428-2300
                                   or
                                   (818) 795-7553

Montgomery Laboratories   (818) 796-9141

Wilson Laboratories   (800) 255-7912
  Kansas residents call: (800) 432-7921

Suburban Water Testing Laboratories (800) 433-6595
  Pennsylvania residents call: (800) 525-6464

Water Test Corporation   (800) 426-8378

National Testing Laboratories   (800) 458-3330

Testing for Chlorine

These suppliers have testing equipment that allows you to find out whether chlorine is getting through your filter into finished water:

Chemetrics
Rte. 28
Calverton, Va. 22016
(800) 356-3072
(703) 788-9026 in Virginia

Hach Chemical Company
Box 389
Loveland, Colo. 80539
(800) 227-4224
(303) 669-3050 in Colorado

LaMotte Chemical Products
Box 329
Chestertown, Md. 21620
(800) 344-3100
(301) 778-3100 in Maryland
FAX: (301) 778-6394

Taylor Chemicals
31 Loveton Circle
Sparks, Md. 21152
(800) 638-4776
FAX: (301) 771-4291

Water Hotline

Safe drinking water hotline
(800) 426-4791
(202) 382-5533 in Washington, D.C.

The hotline was established to explain the Safe Drinking Water Act and its enforcement to the public and to water professionals. EPA specialists are available to answer your questions or refer you to appropriate documents between 8:30 A.M. and 4:30 P.M. EST.

SOURCES OF SUPPLY

Middlemen Services

Nigra Enterprises
5699 Kanan Rd.
Agoura, Calif. 91301
(818) 889-6877
Broker for environmental
systems. Personalized
services to aid consumer in
choosing effective air and
water quality equipment as
well as nontoxic household
products and building
materials.

Air-to-Air Heat Exchangers

Airxchange
401 V.F.W. Dr.
Rockland, Mass. 02370
(617) 871-4816
FAX: (617) 871-3029

Amerix
15 South 15th St.
Fargo, N.D. 58103
(701) 232-4116

Berner Air Products
P.O. Box 5410
New Castle, Pa. 16105
(800) 852-5015
(412) 658-3551 in
Pennsylvania

Des Champs Laboratories
Box 440
East Hanover, N.J. 07936
(201) 884-1460
FAX: (201) 994-4660

EER Products
3536 East 28th St.
Minneapolis, Minn. 55406
(612) 721-4231
FAX: (612) 721-6303

Engineering Development
4850 Northpark Dr.
Colorado Springs,
Colo. 80918
(719) 599-9080

Nutech Energy Systems
124 Newbold Ct.
London, Ontario N6E 1Z7
Canada
(519) 686-0797

Q-Dot Corp.
701 North First St.
Garland, Tex. 75040

Snappy A-D-P
P.O. Box 1168
Detroit Lakes, Minn. 56501
(218) 847-9258

Ventilation Systems

American ALDES
Ventilation Corp.
4539 Northgate Court
Sarasota, Fla. 34234

DEC International
1919 South Stoughton Rd.
Madison, Wis. 53716
(800) 533-7533
(608) 222-3484

Riehs & Riehs
501 George St.
New Bern, N.C. 28560
(919) 636-1615

Therma-Stor Products
Group
Box 8050
Madison, Wis. 53708
(608) 222-3484
(800) 533-7533
FAX: (608) 222-9314

Nontoxic Household Products and Building Materials

AFM Enterprises
1140 Stacy Court
Riverside, Calif. 92507
(714) 781-6860
FAX: (714) 781-6892
Cleansers, water-based
paints, paint strippers,
sealers to stop
formaldehyde emissions,
waxes, polishes, glues,
shampoos.

The Allergy Store
Box 2555

Sebastopol, Calif. 95473
(800) 824-7163
(800) 950-6202 in Calif.
Cleansers, skin-care
products, shampoos.

Baubiologie Hardware
207B 16th St.
Pacific Grove, Calif. 93950
(408) 372-8626
Soaps, cleansers, waxes,
paints, glue.

Beneficial Insectary
14751 Oak Run Rd.
Oak Run, Calif. 96069
(916) 472-3715
Sells parasites that kill
houseflies before they
hatch, reducing the need
for home insecticides.

Bon Ami
Faultless Starch Company
1025 West 8th St.
Kansas City, Mo. 64101
(816) 842-1230
Chlorine-free household
cleanser. Available in most
stores.

Dumond Chemicals
1501 Broadway
New York, N.Y. 10036
(212) 869-6350
Lead-based paint removal
system.

Ecco Bella
6 Provost Square, Suite 602
Caldwell, N.J. 07006
(201) 226-5799
FAX: (201) 226-0991
Cosmetics, household
cleansers, safe pesticides.

Livos Plant Chemistry
2641 Cerrillos Rd.
Santa Fe, N.M. 87501
(800) 621-2591
(505) 988-9111
Paints, adhesives, shellacs,
stains, waxes, art materials,
household cleansers.

Oakmont Industries
44 Oak Street
Newton Upper Falls,
Mass. 02164
(800) 447-2229
FAX: (617) 899-8726
Nontoxic pesticides.

Pace Chem Industries, Inc.
779 LaGrange Ave.
Newbury Park, Calif. 91320
(805) 496-6224
Paints, sealants.

Shaklee Corp.
444 Market St.
San Francisco, Calif. 94111
(800) 544-8860

Sinan Company
Box 181

Suisun City, Calif. 94585
(707) 427-2325
Paints, waxes, soaps.

The Sprout House
40 Railroad Street
Great Barrington,
Mass. 01230
(413) 528-5200
Household cleansers.

Sunrise Lane
780 Greenwich Street
New York, N.Y. 10014
(212) 242-7014
Cosmetics, cleansers, soaps.

AIR PURIFIERS
Electrostatic Air Cleaners

Air Control Industries
213 McLemore St.
Nashville, Tenn. 37203
(615) 242-3448

Air Quality Engineering
3340 Winpark Dr.
Minneapolis, Minn. 55427
(800) 328-0787
(612) 544-4426 in Minnesota
FAX: (612) 544-4013

The Allergy Store
Box 2555
Sebastopol, Calif. 95473
(800) 824-7163
(800) 950-6202 in California

The Environmental
Network
6015 East Commerce,
Suite 430
Irving, Tex. 75063
(214) 550-0808

Honeywell
1985 Douglas Dr., N.
Golden Valley, Minn. 55422
(612) 542-6723

Newtron Products
3874 Virginia Ave.
Cincinnati, Ohio 45227
(800) 543-9149
(513) 561-7373 in Ohio

Permatron Corporation
10134 Pacific Ave.
Franklin Park, Ill. 60131
(800) 882-8012
(312) 678-0314 in Illinois

Summit Hill Laboratories
Navesink, N.J. 07752
(201) 291-3600

Tectronic Products
6500 Badgley Rd.
East Syracuse, N.Y. 13057
(315) 463-0240
FAX: (315) 437-7290

Universal Air Precipitator
Corp.
1500 McCully Rd.
Monroeville, Pa. 15146
(412) 372-0706

HEPA Air Cleaners and Activated Carbon Filters

Airguard Industries
Box 32578
Louisville, Ky. 40232
(502) 969-2304
FAX: (502) 969-2759

Allergen Air Filter
Corporation
5205 Ashbrook
Houston, Tex. 77081
(800) 333-8880

Brian Pure Aire
9307 State Rte. 43
Streetboro, Ohio 44241
(800) 458-5200
(216) 626-5400 in Ohio

Cameron-Yakima Inc.
Box 1554
Yakima, Wash. 98907
(509) 452-6605

Dust Free
Box 454
Royse City, Tex. 75089
(800) 441-1107
(214) 635-9565 in Texas

Envirocaire
747 Bowman Ave.
Hagerstown, Md. 21740
(800) 332-1110
(301) 797-9700 in Maryland

E.L. Foust
Box 105
Elmhurst, Ill. 60125
(800) 225-9549

Mason Engineering and
Designing
242 West Devon Ave.
Bensenville, Ill. 60106
(312) 595-5000

Research Products
1015 East Washington Ave.
Madison, Wis. 53703
(800) 356-9652
(608) 257-8801 in
Wisconsin

3M Filtration Products
76-1W, 3M Center
St. Paul, Minn. 55144
(612) 733-1110

Vitaire
P.O. Box 88
Elmhurst Annex,
N.Y. 11380
(800) 447-4344
(201) 473-2244 in New York

HEPA Vacuum Cleaners
_____

Critical Vacuum Systems
6862 Flying Cloud Dr.
Eden Prairie, Minn. 55344
(800) 328-8322, ext. 582
(612) 829-0836 in Minnesota

Euroclean
907 West Irving Park Rd.
Itasca, Ill. 60143
(800) 323-3553
(312) 773-2111 in Illinois

Healthmore, Inc.
3500 Payne
Cleveland, Oh. 44114
(216) 432-1990 or
(800) 344-1840

NFE International Limited
302 Beeline Dr.
Bensenville, Ill. 60106
(800) 752-2400
(312) 350-1110 in Illinois
FAX: (312) 350-1033

Nilfisk of America
300 Technology Dr.
Malvern, PA 19355
(215) 647-6420

Rexair, Inc.
3221 W. Big Beaver
Suite 200
Troy, Mich. 48084
(313) 643-7222

Vactagon Pneumatic
Systems
25 Power Ave.
Wayne, N.J. 07470
(201) 942-2500

Ion-Exchange Air Cleaners

Air Ion Devices
P.O. Box 5009
Novato, Calif. 94948-5009
(800) 388-4667

WATER PURIFICATION DEVICES

Activated Carbon Filters

Cuno
400 Research Pkwy.
Meriden, Conn. 06950

The Environmental
Network
6015 East Commerce,
Suite 430
Irving, Tex. 75063
(214) 550-0808

Multi-Pure Drinking Water
Systems
9200 Deering Ave.
Chatsworth, Calif. 91311
(818) 341-7577

Reverse-Osmosis Filters

Aquathin Corporation
2800 West Cypress
Creek Blvd.
Fort Lauderdale, Fla. 33309
(305) 977-7997
FAX: (305) 978-6812

General Ecology
151 Sheree Blvd.
Lionville, Pa. 19353
(215) 363-7900
FAX: (215) 363-0412

Distillers

Dupont
Applied Technology
Division
P.O. Box 110
Kennett Square, Pa. 19348

Durastill
875 Brookfield Pkwy.
Rosewell, Ga. 30075
(404) 993-7575

Jordan Chemical Company
P.O. Box 3164
Pikeville, Ky. 41501

Polar Bear Water Distillers
829 Lynnhaven Pkwy.,
Suite 119
Virginia Beach, Va. 23452
(800) 222-7188
(800) 523-6388 in Virginia

Superstill Technology
888 Second Ave.
Redwood City, Calif. 94063
(415) 366-1133

Technical Services Dept.
3M Corporation
3M Center
St. Paul, Minn. 55144
(612) 773-1110

Organic Chemicals Test Kits

Industrial Scientific Corp.
355 Steubenville Pike
Oakdale, Pa. 15071
(412) 758-4353

National Draeger Inc.
Box 120
Pittsburgh, Pa. 15230
(412) 787-8383

Technical Services Dept.
3M Corporation
3M Center
St. Paul, Minn. 55144
(612) 773-1110

Nitrogen Dioxide Test Kits

MDA Scientific
405 Barclay Rd.
Lincolnshire, Ill. 60069
(800) 323-2000

GLOSSARY

adsorption. The process by which contaminants in air or water are physically or chemically attracted to the surface of a solid. Activated carbon captures individual molecules of gases by adsorption.

aerosol. A solid or liquid particle small enough to become suspended in the air. Aerosol cans use compressed gas to dispense a liquid product.

air cleaner. A device that removes contaminants from indoor air. Air-cleaning devices most commonly use mechanical filtration, electrostatic precipitation, or ion generation to purify the air.

air changes per hour. Average number of times within one hour that indoor air is replaced by fresh outdoor air.

allergen. Any substance that produces a hypersensitive, or allergic, reaction in the body. Pollens, mold spores, tobacco smoke, house dust, and airborne chemicals are common allergens.

aquifer. A porous underground formation that contains groundwater. Often found in the voids between particles of sand and gravel or the cracks in shattered bedrock.

asbestos. A naturally occurring family of fibrous minerals that is waterproof, resistant to friction and corrosion, and sound absorbent. Chrysolite asbestos is used in 95 percent of the 3,000 commercial products that contain the mineral. Airborne asbestos fibers are highly toxic.

backdrafting. Reverse airflow down flues or chimneys that allows exhaust gases from combustion appliances to return indoors. Caused by negative air pressure, which results when the outdoor air is insufficient to compensate for the stale air being blown out of a building. Generally associated with tightly sealed houses.

benzo-(a)-pyrene. A tarry organic chemical that pollutes indoor air as the result of incomplete combustion. A known carcinogen.

253

building-related illness. An identifiable affliction that can be traced to a specific pollutant or pollutants inside a building.

carbon monoxide. A colorless, odorless gas created by incomplete combustion. Automobiles, poorly adjusted gas or oil appliances, and portable space heaters, wood stoves, and fireplaces are common sources of the noxious gas.

carcinogen. Any substance capable of causing cancer.

combustion by-products. Any gas, including polynuclear aromatic hydrocarbons, carbon monoxide, and nitrogen dioxide, that is produced by the burning of wood or fossil fuels.

concentration. The amount of a pollutant in a given volume of air.

condensation. The precipitation of airborne water vapor.

contaminant. A substance that is not normally present in clean air or water or one that is present in a greater-than-normal concentration.

cubic feet per minute. A measure of air movement used to rate the relative effectiveness of mechanical ventilation equipment.

dander. Tiny scales from human or animal hair, skin, or feathers.

dust. Bits of solid matter that have been broken into tiny pieces. Road dust is composed primarily of metals including lead, copper, zinc, iron, manganese, chromium, magnesium, and nickel. Household dust commonly contains organic materials such as dust mites, viruses, bacteria, pollens, and dried skin flakes.

effluent. Treated water that is returned to lakes, streams, and aquifers from municipal sewage plants, industrial operations, and household septic tanks.

eutrophication. A process through which a body of water becomes richer in nutrients and lower in dissolved oxygen content, reducing the waterway's ability to support fish. Communities in many parts of the nation have banned phosphate detergents, one source of the excess nutrients that cause eutrophication, in an attempt to reverse the trend.

exfiltration. The passage of interior air from a building through cracks and holes in its envelope.

exhaust air. Stale air that flows out of a house by means of natural or forced ventilation.

formaldehyde. An organic chemical widely used in glues, including those found in plywood, particleboard, paneling, and furniture, and in insulation, carpeting, draperies, and a variety of common household products.

fumes. Smoke, vapor, or gas formed during the combustion process.

gas. A formless liquid that expands to occupy a space or enclosure completely and uniformly. Gas molecules are less than 0.0001 micron in size.

groundwater. Rainwater that collects in an aquifer and supplies 50 percent of the drinking water in the United States.

humidifier fever. A respiratory disease that results in influenzalike symptoms. Also called air conditioner or ventilation fever, it is caused by exposure to toxins emitted by microorganisms that become established in air conditioners or humidifiers.

HVAC system. The centralized heating, ventilation, and air-conditioning system used in a commercial building to regulate temperature, humidity, and air quality.

hypersensitivity pneumonitis. A group of respiratory diseases that involve inflammation of the lungs and are caused by exposure to a biological agent.

infiltration. The passage of outdoor air into a building through cracks in the building's shell and around windows and doors.

microbe. A microorganism, living or dead. Bacteria, viruses, mold, fungi, spores, and pollen are all microbes.

nitrogen dioxide. A gas formed during combustion, especially when gas, oil, or kerosene is burned at high temperatures.

organic chemicals. Molecules that contain carbon as one of their chemical building blocks.

outgassing. The emission of gases such as formaldehyde from building materials into the air as a result of chemical changes.

particulate. Solid or liquid airborne matter that is larger than a single molecule but smaller than 0.5 mm.

pesticides. Family of chemicals used to control undesirable species. Chemicals include insecticides, termiticides, nematocides, herbicides, fungicides, and rodenticides.

pollutant. A contaminant found in concentrations high enough to adversely affect human health or the environment.

polynuclear aromatic hydrocarbons. A group of organic compounds formed by incomplete combustion, which includes benzo-(a)-pyrene.

radon. A gas formed by the natural decay of uranium, which is found in granites, shales, and phosphate-bearing rocks. Within about two weeks of its release, radon decays into a family of radioactive radon daughters that can become lodged in lung tissue and increase the risk of cancer.

recirculated air. Indoor air that passes through an HVAC system to be heated or cooled, then returned through the building. Generally, a small percentage of fresh outdoor air is mixed with the recirculating indoor air.

relative humidity. The ratio of actual airborne water vapor to the maximum the air can potentially hold at a given temperature.

respirable suspended particulates. Bits of airborne matter small enough to be inhaled deep into the lungs yet large enough to become lodged there once they enter.

sick building syndrome. A set of symptoms shared by many building occupants that are not associated with a specific disease or caused by a known pollutant, but which diminish or disappear entirely when building occupants leave.

solvent. A substance that can dissolve another substance. Commonly used chemical solvents include trichloroethylene, xylene, trichloroethane, toluene, and benzene.

surface water. Water contained in lakes, rivers, streams, and reservoirs that provides the source of half the nation's drinking water.

vapor. The gaseous state of a substance that is normally liquid or solid.

ventilation rate. The rate at which fresh outdoor air is introduced to replace stale air in a building through natural or forced ventilation methods. Air changes per hour (ac/h) and cubic feet per minute (cf/m) are two common ways of measuring ventilation rates.

volatile organic compounds. Chemical compounds that contain carbon and evaporate at room temperature.

BIBLIOGRAPHY

OVERVIEW OF INDOOR AIR POLLUTION

Books

Air Quality, by Thad Godish. 1985. (Available from: Lewis Publishers, 121 South Main St., Chelsea, Mich. 48118.)

A technical look at the primary sources and health effects of air pollution. One chapter is devoted specifically to indoor air quality.

Indoor Air Quality, by Beat Meyer. Addison-Wesley Publishing, Reading, Mass. 1983.

In-depth, technical look at the sources and health effects of indoor air pollution.

Indoor Air Quality and Human Health, by Isaac Turiel. Stanford University Press, Stanford, Calif. 1985.

A major reference on the subject.

Indoor Pollutants. National Academy Press. 1981. (Available from: National Technical Information Service, U.S. Department of Commerce, 5285 Port Royal Rd., Springfield, Va. 22161.)

Reviews sources of airborne pollutants, their health effects, and how to control them in the home, workplace, and other public buildings. Makes recommendations for further research.

Reports and Articles

"Controlling Indoor Air Pollution," by Anthony V. Nero, Jr. *Scientific American,* May 1988.

Considers the risks from pollution and discusses the regulation of indoor air.

"Health Effects and Sources of Indoor Air Pollution, Part I and Part II," by Jonathan M. Samet, et al. *American Review of Respiratory Diseases,* 1987, Vols. 136 and 137.

Detailed scholarly analysis of the major pollutants and their health effects.

"Indoor Air Pollution: A Public Health Perspective," by John D. Spengler and Ken Sexton. *Science,* July 1983.

Covers the health risks of specific contaminants and the need to adopt an overall public policy approach to the investigation and control of exposure.

Indoor Air Pollution in Massachusetts. Final Report of the Special Legislative Commission on Indoor Air Pollution. April 1989. (Available from: Office of Senator William B. Golden, Room 416 B, State House, Boston, Mass. 02133.)

258

One of the best nontechnical overviews of the indoor air pollution problem, prepared for the Massachusetts state government. Includes information on specific contaminants as well as public policy recommendations.

"Indoor Air Quality Position Paper." 1987. (Available from: ASHRAE, 1791 Tullie Circle, N.E., Atlanta, Ga. 30329.)

Position paper that outlines the problems of indoor pollution and the professional association's recommendations for reducing it.

"The Inside Story: A Guide to Indoor Air Quality." Office of Air and Radiation, Environmental Protection Agency. (Available from: Environmental Protection Agency, 401 M. St., S.E., Washington, D.C. 20460.)

Readable and informative summary of major pollutants and how to control them.

Newsletters

Indoor Air News. Consumer Federation of America. Periodic. (Available from: Consumer Federation of America, 1424 16th St., N.W., Washington, D.C. 20036.)

Indoor Air Quality Update. Cutter Information Corp. Monthly. (Available from: Cutter Information Corp., 1100 Massachusetts Ave., Arlington, Mass. 02174.)

Indoor Pollution News: The Bi-Weekly Newsletter on Regulation, Legislation, and Litigation. Buraff Publications. Biweekly. (Available from: Bureau of National Affairs, 2445 M St., N.W., Suite 275, Washington, D.C. 20037.)

Congressional Testimony

Legislative hearings before congressional committees provide detailed scientific and anecdotal information about indoor pollution problems. Available from: Superintendent of Documents, Congressional Sales Office, U.S. Government Printing Office, Washington, D.C. 20402 or the relevant subcommittee.

"Indoor Air Quality Act of 1989." Hearing before the Subcommittee on Superfund, Ocean, and Water Protection of the Committee on Environment and Public Works. United States Senate. May 3, 1989.

"Indoor Air Quality Act of 1987." Hearing before the Subcommittee on Environmental Protection of the Committee on Environment and Public Works. United States Senate. November 20, 1987.

"Health Effects of Indoor Air Pollution." Hearing before the Subcommittee on Environmental Protection of the Committee on Environment and Public Works. United States Senate. April 24, 1987.

IN THE HOME

Books

Air-to-Air Heat Exchangers for Houses, by William A. Shurcliff. 1982. (Available from: Brick House Publishing, Box 134, Acton, Mass. 01720.)

Technical discussion of heat-recovery ventilation, humidity, and air-to-air heat exchangers. Thirty-five types of exchangers are described, with a discussion of the advantages and disadvantages given for each one. Heavily illustrated.

The Complete Book of Home Environmental Hazards, by Roberta Altman. Facts on File, New York. 1990.

Complete Trash: The Best Way to Get Rid of Practically Everything Around the House, by Norm Crampton. M. Evans and Co., New York. 1989.

An alphabetized listing of toxic household refuse plus instructions on how to dispose of each item safely.

Healthful Houses: How to Design and Build Your Own, by Clint Good and Debra Lynn Dadd. 1988. (Available from: Guaranty Press, 4720 Montgomery Ln., Suite 1010, Bethesda, Md. 20814.)

How to design a home that uses natural ventilation available on the site, minimizes use of polluting materials, and makes efficient use of energy. Specifications are included for building materials, wiring, plumbing supplies, and HVAC equipment.

The Healthy Home: An Attic-to-Basement Guide to Toxin-Free Living, by Linda Mason Hunter. Rodale Press, Emmaus, Pa. 1989.

A room-by-room guide to possible dangers in the home, from tainted water and polluted air to safety and security hazards, plus ways to eliminate them.

The Healthy House: How to Buy One, How to Build One, How to Cure a "Sick" One, by John Bower. Lyle Stuart, New York. 1989.

A guideline for the homeowner and the would-be homeowner.

Healthy House Catalog, by Environmental Health Watch and Housing Resource Center. 1989. (Available from: Environmental Health Watch, 4115 Bridge Ave., Cleveland, Ohio 44113.)

How to control indoor air pollution. Features extensive source lists for building materials, ventilation equipment, and household products.

Home Ecology, by Karen Christensen. Arlington Books, London. 1989. (Available from: Arlington Books, 15-17 King St., St. James's, London SW1, United Kingdom.)

How to conserve energy and water, recycle, and solve indoor air pollution problems.

Home Heating and Cooling, by Kenneth Winchester. Time-Life Books, Richmond, Va. 1988.

The basics of HVAC systems and electrical controls aimed at helping the homeowner perform maintenance and repairs. Tells how to replace filters and clean blower motors, air conditioner condensate pans, and humidifier evaporator pads and when to seek professional help. Heavily illustrated.

House Dangerous: Indoor Pollution in Your Home and Office—and What You Can Do about It, by Ellen J. Greenfield. Vintage, New York. 1987.

Takes readers on a tour of the home and workplace to identify sources of pollution and provide ways to deal with them.

The Nontoxic Home: Protecting Yourself and Your Family from Everyday Toxics and Health Hazards, by Debra Lynn Dadd. Jeremy P. Tarcher, Inc., Los Angeles. 1986.

Describes safe alternatives to everyday cleaning, personal care, and household products.

Your Home, Your Health and Well-Being, by David Rousseau, W.J. Rea, M.D., and Jean Enwright. Ten Speed Press, Berkeley, Calif. 1988.

How indoor air quality, light, color, and sound all affect health and how to design a healthy home. Includes room-by-room design plans and a look at ventilation and other building systems.

Reports and Articles

"Air-to-Air Heat Exchangers." "Indoor Air Quality." Fact sheets on combustion, formaldehyde, moisture, particles, and radon. (Available from: Energy Library, Washington State Energy Office, 809 Legion Way, S.E., FA-11, Olympia, Wash. 98504.)

Fact sheets and pamphlets on a number of residential home air quality issues. Publications on energy conservation are also available.

"A Citizen's Guide to Pesticides." (Available from: Office of Pesticides and Toxic Substances, Environmental Protection Agency, Washington, D.C. 20460.)

How to use pesticides safely and reduce your exposure.

"Heat Recovery Ventilation for Housing: Air-to-Air Heat Exchangers." Department of Energy. February 1984. (Available from: Department of Energy, Washington, D.C. 20585.)

Everything a homeowner needs to know about choosing and installing an air-to-air heat exchanger.

"Home Ventilating Guide." Published annually by the Home Ventilating Institute. (Available from: Home Ventilating Institute, 30 West University Dr., Arlington Heights, Ill. 60004.)

A directory of ventilating products, including ratings of air delivery and relative noise levels.

"Issue Backgrounder: Energy Efficient New Homes and Indoor Pollutants," August 1987. "Home Weatherization and Indoor Air Pollutants," November

1984. (Available from: Bonneville Power Administration, Public Involvement Office, P.O. Box 12999, Portland, Ore. 97212.)

Excellent overviews of indoor air pollution problems in the home and how to combat them without losing energy efficiency.

"Moisture Control in Homes." 1987. (Available from Conservation and Renewable Energy Inquiry and Referral Service, U.S. Department of Energy, Box 8900, Silver Spring, Md. 20907.)

Pamphlet covering the basics of moisture-related problems and what to do about them, including the use of air-to-air heat exchangers. Lists further sources on the subject.

"Recommendations for the Use of Residential Air-Cleaning Devices in the Treatment of Allergic Respiratory Diseases," by Dr. Harold S. Nelson, et al. *Journal of Allergy and Clinical Immunology*, October 1988.

An overview of air purification devices.

"The Ten Most Asked Questions About Home Ventilation," by G. Granson. *Family Handyman*, January 1986.

"Viruses and Indoor Air Pollution," by Dr. Robert B. Couch. Bulletin, New York Academy of Medicine. December 1981. (Available from: Dr. Robert B. Couch, Baylor College of Medicine, 1200 Moursund Ave., Houston, Tex. 77030.)

How viruses contaminate indoor air and cause disease.

OFFICES AND OTHER PUBLIC BUILDINGS

Books

Office Hazards: How Your Job Can Make Your Sick, by Joel Makower. Tilden Press, Washington, D.C. 1981.

About the hazards of working in an office, including pollution, radiation, high noise levels, and stress, and how to reduce them.

Office Work Can Be Dangerous to Your Health, by Jeanne Stellman and Mary Sue Hennifin. Pantheon Books, New York. 1983.

A handbook of office health and safety hazards and what can be done to protect yourself. Includes material on indoor air pollution.

Reports and Articles

"Air Contaminants—Permissible Exposure Limits." Title 29, Code of Federal Regulations. Occupational Safety and Health Administration. (Available from: Superintendent of Documents, U.S. Government Printing Office, Washington, D.C. 20402.)

Federal standards for maximum contaminant concentration levels in industrial settings. Most OSHA standards are considered too high for long-term exposure in office buildings, but they provide a useful guideline.

"Guidance for Indoor Air Quality Investigations." (Available from: Hazards Evaluation and Technical Assistance Branch, National Institute for Occupational Safety and Health, 4676 Columbia Pkwy., Cincinnati, Ohio 45226.)

Detailed description of how to investigate complaints in a commercial building and how to implement corrective measures.

"Indoor Air Facts." (Available from: U.S. Environmental Protection Agency, 401 M St., S.E., Washington, D.C. 20460.)

A series of papers issued by the Environmental Protection Agency, including "EPA and Indoor Air Quality," "Indoor Air Quality Implementation Plan," "Ventilation and Air Quality in Offices," and "Sick Buildings."

"Indoor Air Pollution in Offices and Other Non-Residential Buildings." *Journal of Environmental Health*, January–February 1986. (Available from: Thad Godish, Ph.D., Director, Indoor Air Quality Research Laboratory, Ball State University, Department of Natural Resources, Muncie, Ind. 47306.)

Good background on sources and consequences of workplace pollution.

"Indoor Air Quality: Maryland Public Schools." November 1987. (Available from: Allen C. Abend, Director, Office of School Facilities, Maryland State Department of Education, 200 West Baltimore St., Baltimore, Md. 21201.)

Excellent overview of indoor air quality in public buildings.

"Liability for Indoor Air Pollution in the Workplace," by Laurence S. Kirsch, Esq. (Available from: Laurence S. Kirsch, Esquire, Cadwalader, Wickersham & Taft, 1333 New Hampshire Ave., N.W., Washington, D.C. 20036.)

Reviews the precedents and potential of liability suits stemming from indoor pollution complaints against employers, building managers, and others.

"Systematic Investigation Needed for Tight Building Syndrome Complaints." *Occupational Health and Safety*, May 1987.

Emphasizes the need to respond to complaints from white-collar workers.

"Ventilation for Acceptable Indoor Air Quality." ASHRAE Standard 62-1989. (Available from: ASHRAE, 1791 Tullie Circle, N.E., Atlanta, Ga. 30329.)

Voluntary guideline for determining appropriate ventilation rates in commercial buildings.

SOURCES ON SPECIFIC CONTAMINANTS

Asbestos

"Asbestos in Buildings: What Owners and Managers Should Know." (Available from: Safe Buildings Alliance, Suite 1200, 655 15th St., N.W., Washington, D.C. 20005.)

Report summarizing current asbestos regulations and appropriate assessment and response actions. Seeks to downplay the risks of asbestos.

"Asbestos in the Home." U.S. Consumer Product Safety Commission. 1982. (Available from: Superintendent of Documents, U.S. Government Printing Office, Washington, D.C. 20402.)

Good primer on where asbestos might be found in the home and what to do about it.

"Living with Asbestos," by Dr. Ronald G. Crystal. *Medical and Health Annual.* Encyclopedia Britannica. 1986.

History of asbestos use and its link to human health.

Cigarette Smoke

Clearing the Air: Perspectives on Environmental Tobacco Smoke, edited by Robert D. Tollison. 1988. (Available from: Lexington Books, 125 Spring St., Lexington, Mass. 02173.)

Goes well beyond its subtitle to confront the technical, legal, and political aspects of indoor air pollution.

"A Decision Maker's Guide to Reducing Smoking at the Worksite." 1985. (Available: Office of Disease Prevention and Health Promotion, 2132 Switzer Building, 330 C St., S.W., Washington, D.C. 20201.)

How to develop and implement workplace smoking policies.

Smoking and Health Review. Action on Smoking and Health. (Available from ASH, 2013 H St., N.W., Washington, D.C. 20006.)

Newsletter dedicated to reducing or eliminating smoking in public places. ASH has many other fact sheets, including "The Effects of Involuntary Smoking" and "Non-Smoking Sections in Restaurants."

Surgeon General's Report on Smoking. Annual. *Smoking and Health Bulletin.* Bi-monthly. "The Health Consequences of Involuntary Smoking." A report of the Surgeon General. 1986. (Available from: Office on Smoking and Health, Center for Health Promotion and Education, Parklawn Building, Room 1-10, 5600 Fishers Ln., Rockville, Md. 20857.)

Radon

"A Citizen's Guide to Radon: What It Is and What to Do about It." "Radon Reduction Methods: A Homeowner's Guide." "Removal of Radon from Household Water." (Available from: Office of Radiation Programs, Radon Programs, Environmental Protection Agency, 401 M St., S.W., Washington, D.C. 20460.)

Booklets detailing effective techniques for eliminating radon from the home.

"Backgrounder: Understanding Indoor Radon." (Available from: Bonneville Power Administration, Public Involvement Office, P.O. Box 12999, Portland, Ore. 97212.)

Good summary of major radon concerns.

"Citizen's Guide to Radon Home Test Kits." (Available from: Public Citizen, Box 19404, Washington, D.C. 20036.)

A poster-size guide to commercial radon testing, including an evaluation of specific manufacturers.

"Radon Detectors: How to Find Out If Your House Has a Radon Problem." *Consumer Reports*, July 1987.

A good overview of the radon problem, plus testing methods and solutions.

Radon: A Homeowner's Guide to Detection and Control, by Bernard Cohen. 1987. (Available from: Consumer Reports Books, 540 Barnum Ave., Bridgeport, Conn. 06608.)

An overview of the radon problem, including where radon is found, how it can be measured, and how risks can be lessened. Includes *Consumer Reports'* recommendations and ratings of the leading radon detectors on the market.

"Radon Exposure: Human Health Threat." Congressional hearing before the Subcommittee on Health and the Environment of the Committee on Energy and Commerce. United States House of Representatives. November 5, 1987. (Available from: Superintendent of Documents, Congressional Sales Office, U.S. Government Printing Office, Washington, D.C. 20402.)

"Radon Gas Issues." Joint congressional hearing before the Subcommittees on Environmental Protection and Superfund and Environmental Oversight of the Committee on Environment and Public Works. United States Senate. April 2, 1987. (Available from: Superintendent of Documents, Congressional Sales Office, U.S. Government Printing Office, Washington, D.C. 20402.)

Radon: The Invisible Threat, by Michael LaFavore. Rodale Press, Emmaus, Pa. 1987.

Everything a consumer needs to know about what radon is, where it is found, and how you can protect yourself from its dangers.

"Radon Pollution Control Act of 1987." Congressional hearing before the Subcommittee on Transportation, Tourism, and Hazardous Materials of the Committee on Energy and Commerce. United States House of Representatives. April 23, 1987. (Available from: Superintendent of Documents, Congressional Sales Office, U.S. Government Printing Office, Washington, D.C. 20402.)

WATER

Books

But Not a Drop to Drink! The Life-Saving Guide to Good Water, by Steve Coffel. Rawson Associates, New York. 1989.

Comprehensive overview on the growing water crisis and how to make sure that your household water is safe.

Cadillac Desert, by Marc Reiner. Viking, New York. 1986.

The irrigation used to make agriculture possible in the arid West is the "Cadillac" described here. Reiner explains how irrigation taints drinking water with salts and pesticides.

Drinking Water and Health. Safe Drinking Water Committee of the National Academy of Sciences. Vol. 1, 1977; Vols. 2 and 3, 1980; Vol. 4, 1982; Vol. 5, 1983; Vol. 6, 1986; Vols. 7 and 8, 1987. (Available from: National Academy Press, 2101 Constitution Ave., N.W., Washington, D.C. 20418.)

Periodic reports on the health effects of toxic substances found in drinking water, issued by the National Academy of Sciences, as mandated by the Safe Drinking Water Act.

Future Water, by John R. Scheaffer and Leonard A. Stevens. William A. Morrow, New York. 1983.

Documents the promise of "circular management" of water resources, which uses natural processes to remove and use nutrients and other contaminants in waste water, cleaning up the water for reuse in the process.

A Life of Its Own, by Robert Gottlieb. Harcourt Brace Jovanovich, New York. 1988.

A provocative analysis of the politics and power of water which suggests that quality is being sacrificed in the rush to provide ever-growing quantities of water to a thirsty nation.

Troubled Water, by Jonathan King. Rodale Press, Emmaus, Pa. 1985.

Documents the contamination of drinking water by pesticides, toxic wastes, emissions from military installations, and pollutants generated in the treatment process.

Periodicals

"Groundwater Monitor." (Available from: Business Publishers, Inc., 951 Pershing Dr., Silver Spring, Md. 20910.)

Bi-weekly newsletter reporting on legislation, regulations, court decisions, state and local actions, new technology, and business news affecting groundwater.

Journal of the American Water Works Association. (Available from: AWWA, 6666 West Quincy Ave., Denver, Colo. 80235.)

A monthly magazine on water supply management and research, published by the association of water supply professionals. Other publications relating to drinking water quality are also available.

U.S. Water News. (Available from: U.S. Water News, 230 Main St., Halstead, Kans. 67056.)

An excellent monthly newspaper devoted to water, its pollution and use, published jointly by *U.S. Water News* and the Freshwater Foundation.

Western Water. (Available from: Water Education Foundation, 717 K St., Suite 517, Sacramento, Calif. 95814.)

Bi-monthly magazine focusing on California water quality, but of interest to readers in all parts of the country.

Reports and Articles

"Acid Deposition: Trends, Relationships and Effects." National Research Council. May 1986. (Available from: National Academy Press, 2101 Constitution Ave., N.W., Washington, D.C. 20418.)

Report summarizing the process by which industrial emissions, especially sulfur dioxide, cause acid rain, which in turn increases the acidity of lakes and streams. Also identifies the parts of the country with the most acidic rainfall.

"America's Clean Water." (Available from: Association of State and Interstate Water Pollution Control Administrators, 444 North Capitol St., N.W., Washington, D.C. 20001. (202) 624-7782.)

A series of pamphlets that summarize the progress made in cleaning up the nation's water.

"Water-Quality Trends in the Nation's Rivers." (Available from: U.S. Government Printing Office, N. Capitol and H Streets, Washington, D.C. 20401.)

U.S. Geological Survey study of water quality trends in the nation's rivers summarizes the results of monitoring at 300 locations on U.S. rivers conducted between 1974 and 1981.

"Water: Rethinking Management in an Age of Scarcity" and "Conserving Water: The Untapped Alternative," by Sandra Postel. (Available from: Worldwatch Institute, 1776 Massachusetts Ave., N.W., Washington, D.C. 20036.)

Examines new ways of using and thinking about water resources to improve the supply and quality of drinking water without curtailing irrigated agriculture.

"You and Your Drinking Water." *EPA Journal*, Vol. 12, No. 7. September 1986. (Available from: Office of Public Affairs, U.S. Environmental Protection Agency, Washington, D.C. 20460.)

Primer on drinking water, including the treatment process, how water gets contaminated, and what's being done about it.

CHECKLIST TO INDOOR POLLUTION

What pollution hazards are most commonly found in the

What should I know if I am undertaking renovations at home or buying new furniture?

What else should I consider when building a new house or an addition?

What should I know if I want to conserve energy while preventing poor air quality?

Shortness of breath, 23–24
Eye irritations, 76–77, 78–79
Upper respiratory tract infections, 40–41, 76–77, 80, 82–83
Allergic reactions, 23–24, 37–38, 40–41

What contaminants can cause cancer? 133–38, 170, 172
How can I tell if I am suffering from sick building syndrome? 155

What are the most common household and workplace sources of
Asbestos, 21–23, 25
Formaldehyde, 29–31, 32
Volatile organic compounds, 36–37, 39, 40–41
Radon, 49–50, 51
Biological agents, 65–66, 67
Combustion by-products, 75–76, 78, 79–80, 81

What are the health hazards of
Asbestos, 23–24
Formaldehyde, 31, 33
Volatile organic compounds, 37–38, 40–41
Radon, 51–53
Biological agents, 66, 68
Combustion by-products, 76–77, 78–79, 80, 82–83

How can I reduce the presence of
Asbestos, 26–28
Formaldehyde, 34, 35
Volatile organic compounds, 42, 46
Radon, 56–65
Biological agents, 69, 74
Combustion by-products, 85–88

How can I test the indoor air at home or in the workplace for
Asbestos, 26
Formaldehyde, 34
Volatile organic compounds, 41–42
Radon, 53–55
Biological agents, 69
Combustion by-products, 83–84

INDEX